W9-BKE-895

ETHICS IN
DEAF EDUCATION

ETHICS IN
DEAF EDUCATION

Edited by
Rod G. Beattie

ACADEMIC PRESS

San Diego   London   Boston   New York   Sydney   Tokyo   Toronto

Academic Press
A Harcourt Science and Technology Company
525 B Street, Suite 1900, San Diego, California 92101-4495, USA
http://www.academicpress.com

Academic Press
Harcourt Place, 32 Jamestown Road, London NW1 7BY, UK
http://www.academic press.com

Library of Congress Catalog Card Number: 2001092472

International Standard Book Number: 0-12-083522-3

PRINTED IN THE UNITED STATES OF AMERICA
01   02   03   04   05   06   SB   9   8   7   6   5   4   3   2   1

DEDICATION

Books should be dedicated to someone or something since it is a tradition—
especially books on serious topics—but then maybe not. The decision, however,
on who or what is difficult. Editors and authors, I suppose, in thinking of an
appropriate "who" look for an individual or maybe a group of people who made a
difference, contributed, supported, or is, are, or were loved. What a daunting task!
Perhaps so many! And furthermore, the difference-makers, contributors, supporters, or beloved may not be as giving, generous, gracious, gallant, or gentle—if
they see another's name on the dedication before or in place of theirs. Yes, select-
ing a "who" is difficult, and as everyone knows—in the extreme—public
announcements of favorites have caused wars. If I must choose a who, perhaps it
is best that I dedicate this work to those I apply my favorite pet names of beautiful, handsome, girl, boy, lass, lad, mate, and sweatpea. Or to those I sign the bot-
tom of my correspondence with "love"—for then they shall know who they are.

When who proves too difficult, I suspect, dedication writers fall back to the
safety of a what—an entity—something physical. Personally though, I do not
think a "what" is any easier. At least not in the complex world known as education
of the deaf and hearing impaired. Historically, cooperation, tolerance, open-mindedness, achievement, standing would make poor selection criteria, unless one is
looking for a short list to draw from. Perhaps something ephemeral like diversity
is a thought. It would leave the readers with the option to take it as they wish.
Some will surely think that my tongue was planted securely in epithelial tissue,
whereas others would take the moral high ground, and think the best of me.

Yes, diversity of pet names and signed love—I like that. I dedicated this book
to these.

CONTENTS

1

INTRODUCTION AND OVERVIEW

ROD G. BEATTIE

PART I

FROM BIRTH TO THREE YEARS

2

ETHICAL CONSIDERATIONS IN THE DEMOGRAPHY OF DEAFNESS

JEROME D. SCHEIN

3

DEAFNESS, SCIENCE, TECHNOLOGY, AND ETHICS

DES POWER

4

MOTHER TONGUE/FIRST LANGUAGE

DEENA M. MARTIN, MICHAEL RODDA, AND SUSANNE MARTIN

5

ETHICS OF ASSESSMENT

ELEANOR STEWART AND KATHRYN RITTER

PART II

FROM THREE TO SIX YEARS

6

EQUALITY, EXCELLENCE, AND PARENTAL CHOICE IN EDUCATION OF DEAF AND HARD OF HEARING CHILDREN IN ISRAEL: ETHICS AND BALANCING INDIVIDUAL, GROUP, AND NATIONAL AGENDAS

AMATZIA WEISEL

7

EDUCATIONAL PLACEMENT

WENDY MCCRACKEN

8

CURRICULUM CONSIDERATIONS

GREGORY R. LEIGH

9

ETHICS AND THE PREPARATION OF
TEACHERS OF THE DEAF

DAVID A. STEWART

10

Thoughts and Projections

Rod G. Beattie

ACKNOWLEDGMENTS

To my parents and brother for unconditional love and support given while only shaking their head quietly from great distances.

To the contributing authors for being keen at the beginning and working hard to keep up the emotional energy for the long haul.

To my colleagues at Renwick College and the Royal Institute for Deaf and Blind Children for putting up with the curmudgeon that I am.

To Laura Parker, Sales Representative, Electronic Publishing, Academic Press, for being a great facilitator and an interesting seat-mate on a long flight.

To Mark Zadrozny, Senior Editor at Academic Press, for supporting and tolerating the quirky nature of academic editors and writers.

To Neil, Frank, Tim, Nat, Kirby, Jayne, and Liz because you heard me whinge the longest and the loudest.

CONTRIBUTORS

Numbers in parentheses indicate pages on which the authors' contributions begin

Rod G. Beattie (1, 185) Renwick College, Royal Institute for Deaf and Blind Children, North Rocks, NSW 2151, Australia.

Gregory R. Leigh (143) Renwick College, Royal Institute for Deaf and Blind Children, North Rocks, NSW 2151, Australia.

Deena M. Martin (47) Department of Educational Psychology, Univesity of Alberta, Edmonton, AB T6G 2G5, Canada.

Susanne Martin (47) Department of Educational Psychology, University of Alberta, Edmonton AB T6G 2G5, Canada.

Wendy McCracken (119) Centre for Audiology, Education of the Deaf, and Speech Pathology, University of Manchester, Manchester M13 9PL, United Kingdom.

Des Power (33) Centre for Deafness Studies and Faculty of Education, Griffith University, Brisbane, QLD 4111, Australia.

Kathryn Ritter (67) Department of Audiology and Communication Disorders, Glenrose Rehabilitation Hospital, Edmonton, AB T5G 0B7, Canada

Michael Rodda (47) Department of Educational Psychology, University of Alberta, Edmonton, AB T6G 2G5, Canada.

Jerome D. Schein (21) 1703 Andros Isle, Coconut Creek, Florida 33066.

Michael Steer (xiii) Renwick College, Royal Institute for Deaf and Blind Children, North Rocks, NSW 2151, Australia.

David A. Stewart (167) Michigan State University, East Lansing, Michigan 48824.

Eleanor Stewart (67) 5917 90A Avenue, Edmonton, AB TGB OR1, Canada.

Amatzia Weisel (93) School of Education, Tel Aviv University, Ramat Aviv, Tel Aviv 69978, Israel.

PREFACE

The degree of importance for a book on ethics concerning education and deaf[1] children and their family is unknown. I personally believe it is or should be very important—make that of the highest order! I have thought about the topic of ethics and educational practices for children with hearing losses for a long time. It was probably 15 years ago that I started with an envelope in my desk drawer for topical bits and pieces. Later, the material in this envelope expanded to a series of folders in a filing cabinet—perhaps not as neat and thoughtfully organized as it should have been.

As the folders filled, I started constructing rough outlines for myself. I developed these outlines so that I could file and record relevant information as I happened across it, thought of an idea, had an insight, heard of a problem, or experienced an interesting ethical dilemma. I also started making comments on these outlines about missing information and questions I had. I started all this because I thought it was important to educate myself. I also thought I could better serve teachers-in-training—a role that pays the bills and one I generally see as my most important work. I take some satisfaction that some of the outline titles have a direct lineage to the final chapters in this book written by my contributing authors.

I feel it is important that readers realize that I do not have a degree in ethics. Nor can I even say that I took a focused course in ethics as part of a university degree. Certainly, I remember topics in undergraduate and graduate courses that discussed "classic cases" like the Milgram and Zimbardo studies. My knowledge, however, remains between the levels of a dabbler and perhaps a journeyman with a reasonable amount of experience. The contributing authors, most of whom have decades of professional experience in the field of deafness, likely have more formal training in ethics than I—for it would be difficult to have less.

I will honestly admit my first extended experiences with ethics concerned filling in ethics-review forms for thesis and dissertation research. Later, this experience grew to include the ethics review requirements for research applications with hospitals, universities, and different government agencies. Eventually, I took a seat on department and institutional research and ethics review committees. Unfortunately, little of the committee experience is reflected in the focus of this book. Certainly the four principles approach to ethical practice in research— respect for patient autonomy, beneficience, non-maleficence, and justice—have not been forgotten. So yes, the narrow world of research does have connections to the real world of education and life.

In eagerness then, I offer you two things. I offer first the foreword written by my colleague Dr. Michael Steer, Senior Lecturer in Vision Impairments at Renwick College. This foreword discusses ethics and special education. It provides a wider context, something I found helpful—I trust others will appreciate it as well. Second, I offer you this book on ethics and deaf education focusing on the child's early years. I am sure that each of the contributing authors will pique your interest in the topic in unique ways. I know the material they wrote had that effect on me. I also ask the reader to consider the authors' dilemmas. I am sure each looked for a forerunning model for support. I suspect, like my own efforts, they were unsuccessful. The common comment "this was very difficult to write" was perhaps a reflection of their unsuccessful search. From these comments, I realized that our work would be better described as a start not a finish. With this thought in mind, I urge the readers to start with us as well by reading on.

NOTES

[1] Variation may be found throughout this book on the capitalization of the first letter of the word "deaf." Beginning the word with a capital letter is a convention typically used to signify persons with a hearing loss who participate in and identify with a specific cultural/linguistic group who use a natural sign language. In contrast, uncapitalized use of the word deaf tends to be used more inclusively and is often used to describe an individual's audiological status instead of participation in a cultural/linguistic group. Because interpretation and use of this convention is not universal and the contributing authors are from five different countries, "big-D/little-d" usage may differ across chapters. I will say that I made an editorial effort to achieve consistency.

SERVICE PROVISION TO PEOPLE WITH DISABILITIES: A DEONTOLOGICAL PERSPECTIVE

MICHAEL STEER

Some insight into the ethics of service provision is necessary for those wishing to more fully comprehend the current situation of individuals with disabilities, particularly sensory disabilities in western-style, developed economies. The manner in which societies think about and have generally perceived and treated people with disabilities has an important impact on modern society. This is because presently it is widely held that the ethic that governs the way a society treats its most disadvantaged people, to some extent reflects that society's maturity. Ethics is of course, the branch of philosophy that focuses on the study of moral behavior. It is primarily concerned with examining principles and methods of establishing the ways we should act in morally-laden situations.

When considering the ethics of service provision to people with sensory disabilities, there are different points of view that influence the ethical decision-making process. Two common perspectives are (1) the teleological or consequentialist and (2) the deontological. It is the latter perspective that provides the focus of this preface.

A denotological ethic starts from an assumption that a person's motive or intention for acting is what is important in making ethical judgments. When someone who takes a deontological perspective makes an ethical judgment about a situation, it is the motive or intention of the participants that is judged. When someone taking a deontological perspective attempts to determine the ways we should act, he or she focuses on establishing the primary duties of participants in moral contexts. Such duties might include, for example, doing no harm or respecting autonomy. These types of factors are essential to an understanding of current human service provision since the behavior of human service organizations affects a great many people with sensory impairments who might generally be thought at risk of societal disadvantage.

The manner in which a particular society thinks about people with sensory disabilities, as Cocks and Stehlik (1995) have pointed out, strongly influences their treatment. In turn, the way that people with sensory disabilities are treated strongly influences the manner in which society thinks about them. This circular pattern generates a self-fulfilling prophecy. If, for example, people who are vision or hearing impaired are predominantly viewed by society as ill or defective, then they will be treated within service systems that function as health-care delivery agents. If members of the public see many people with sensory disabilities treated in hospital-like or clinical settings, the initial perception of sickness and defectiveness is strengthened. An outcome of their treatment is that the people with sensory disabilities are likely to internalize their experiences and eventually think of themselves as sick or defective when they are not.

Alternatively, if people with sensory disabilities are widely held to be humans with potential for growth and development and belonging with their families and friends in their home communities, then services are likely to be provided that support related outcomes. The social roles in which people with disabilities (sensory or otherwise) are cast, ultimately shape personal and service outcomes. The American social scientist Wolfensberger (1992) presents an interesting schemata on the historical roles played by people with disabilities. These various role perceptions, for example, viewing a person with a disability as an object of ridicule, a perpetual child, or a burden on society, are universal influences on the social value of those so perceived. These types of perception must be fully understood in order to comprehend the morality underpinning current patterns of service provision to individuals with disabilities.

AN IMPORTANT PARADIGM SHIFT

The history of service provision to people who are deaf or hearing impaired can be obtained from a relatively large number of reputable authors, typically, for example, from Moores (1996). Similarly, the history of services for people who are blind or vision impaired, typically from Kelley and Gale (1998).

Over the past 40 years, many nations in the western (developed) world have gradually realized that their governments need to invest more energy in ensuring that all citizens receive equal treatment and a just share of society's benefits. This realization has been generally reflected in both law and policy (Gooding, 1994). It has also generally been reflected in gradual public attitude change and in the progressively increasing demands being made on such human service systems as schools, legal and medical offices, parks and recreation facilities, transportation systems, employment services, and consumer goods outlets. The public policy debate in many countries at the opening years of the third millennium is no longer whether or not people with sensory and other forms of disability are entitled to services. It is rather, on the ways in which the needs of such individuals can be met fairly and equitably. The underpining motive for this focus upon equality and justice in the treatment of those at risk of societal devaluation can possibly be attributed to the gradual and wide adoption by Westernized society of the broad Judeo-Christian ethic.

An early outcome of the policy debate has been a growing recognition by decision makers that traditional approaches to human service provision have not been, and are not structured to respond adequately to the needs of people with disabilities and their families. Initiatives over the past 30 years have been taken to discover and implement alternative service provision approaches—approaches that either change or replace the existing system structures and relationship. These changes then, enable others to serve individuals in ways consistent with the emerging changes in perspective on the rights of people who have disabilities.

Some of the concepts and service system developments that have emerged over the past 30 years are derived from the widely held belief that a very large number of people with disabilities are able to live as full, contributing members of society in the community. New-look services by placement in one or other of the programs that were traditionally provided for the clients of their particular category (e.g., placement in segregated schools, sheltered workshops, residential units, and nursing homes). The new ethic is predicated on the notion that, if society is to empower people with disabilities to live as full participants within the community, some critically important links missing from our traditional social service systems need to be present.

The broad category "disability" is, regarding human service policy development, easy to use, but difficult to deal with because it covers people of all ages and both genders whose disadvantages may arise from intellectual, physical, sensory, and psychiatric causes, or some mixture of causes. For those with sensory impairments, the disability may be permanent or temporary. If this is so, by implication then, it is also possible to regard able-bodiedness as a temporary condition.

Regarding the current status of service provision, the western mass media provide the local community with daily stories that reveal the exhausting ongoing struggle for simple services, self-respect, and basic rights violations experienced by citizens who may be sensory impaired. For example, there are instances of agencies renting particular buildings for conferences, knowing that the facilities are inaccessible or dangerous to blind or deaf people; taxi drivers abusing people whose absence of sight, or whose dependence on a guide dog they find in some way strange or threatening; residents of certain affluent communities taking legal action against the disabled residents of small group homes in their neighborhoods; parents losing custody battles because of their impairment. So much, then, for the behavioral backdrop against which the current ethic of care is displayed (Conway, Bergin, & Thornton, 1996).

In discussing use of the term "disability" as a category and as the source of discourse, it is likely, as Fulcher (1989) has pointed out, that traditional service provision practices in many so-called developed countries have constructed "disability" as a marginal state of dependence, poverty, unemployment, and denial of citizenship rights. A large part of the lives of elderly people who are blind or deaf, it might be argued, is influenced by regulations imposed by such professional groups as medical practitioners and specialized care systems workers. These various practices tend to construct social exclusion rather than inclusion. A consideration of practices surrounding people with significant sensory disabilities suggests that those so categorized are widely considered as members of an oppressed class of under citizen.

HUMAN SERVICE SYSTEM COMPONENTS

Several human service planners, in particular Wolfensberger (1992), have proposed that the systems set in place by society's private and public sectors to serve and support people with disabilities, whether the consumers' disabilities are physical, intellectual, emotional, or sensory in nature, should, in design resemble a three-legged milking stool. The human services edifice that is erected should rest upon a three-columned foundation consisting of the following essential elements. First, a legislated base. Second, an appropriate human service philosophy or ideology, and third, an array of service provision options that are comprehensive, coordinated, and community-based.

A Legislated Base

The formalization of the parameters of human services philosophy and practice into law is, as Sage and Burrello (1994) have pointed out, the end result of factors related to definitional terminology, philosophical beliefs, history, and local tradition. Actions of our various legislatures and courts are to a large degree reflections of the ethics that motivate what particular societies are ready to accept, believe, and stand behind.

While lawmakers have sometimes led the community to new understandings of the "common good," they must lead from a position that is not too far ahead of the majority. Legal foundations are, therefore, the official codification of the approximate will of the people.

It is likely that the United Nations Universal Declaration of Human Rights of 1948 was the milestone at the beginning of an era in which all participant UN member states were required to take measures that would respect the rights of their citizens. Subsequently for many developed nations, the major legal, social, and administrative frameworks that have guided service provision to people with disabilities owe much to the Universal Declaration and its subsequent Declaration on the Rights of Disabled Persons in 1975. This declaration obliges signatory nations to ensure that people with disabilities have the right to protection from discrimination; to be treated with respect; to have access to education, training, and employment. It also ensures that people with disabilities have the right to have relationships—a social and a family life, and to receive assistance to enable them to become as independent as possible in all aspects of life.

Human rights for Australians with disabilities, like citizens of other nations, have been effected through incorporation of the UN principles into federal and state law. Ideally, major national legislation reflecting an ethic of human rights promotion is passed first. This tool gives the federal government the power to provide monetary grants to the regional authorities for service provision purposes. It also permits the federal government to promulgate regulations specifying the aims and principles to be followed by states and territorial governments when providing services under the Act. Further, all subsequent governments that are recipients of resources under the Act are required to pass complementary legislation confirming the aims and principles of the federal Act (Cibinel & Kiwanuka, 1998).

The deontological nature of the ethics which motivated the statement of principles and the application, or intent of those principles, can, for example, be readily appreciated through an examination of the preamble to the 1993 New South Wales Disability Services Act.

> Persons with disabilities have the same basic human rights as other members of Australian society. They also have the rights to ensure that their specific needs are met. Their rights, which apply irrespective of the nature, origin, type or degree of disability. (NSW Office of Disability, 1994, p. 1)

The 1993 Act further asserts that persons with disabilities have the "inherent right" to respect for their human dignity and worth, to live in and be part of the community, and to realize their individual capacities for physical, social, emotional, and intellectual development. The Act's principles also reinforce the claim that people with disabilities have the same rights as other Australians. They deserve to have services that will facilitate the achieving of a reasonable quality of life. They may choose their own lifestyle while having access to information to allow informed choice that is provided in an appropriate manner relative to their disability and cultural background. Their rights include receiving services in a way that imposes the least restriction to their rights and opportunities. They may also pursue grievances about services without fearing service withdrawal or provider recriminations. And most fundamentally, the "persons with disabilities have the right to protection from neglect, abuse and exploitation" (NSW Office of Disability, 1994, p. 1).

The application of the outlined principles can be appreciated in clause 2 of the same legislation. Here, the Act's sub-clauses state that services and programs of service must be designed and administered so that the underpinning principles of the Act are met. In the New South Wales legislation, used here as an example of "typical" Australian State legislation, a total of 16 points is listed—each carrying the goal of supporting independence, promoting integration, avoiding human rights violations, and ensuring ethical treatment.

In addition to the 1986 Act mentioned previously, the Australian Commonwealth and other nations have enacted legislation to give effect to other international treaty obligations (Fletcher, 1995); for example: The Human Rights and

Equal Opportunity Commission Act (1986), Racial Discrimination Act (1975), Sex Discrimination Act (1984), and the Disability Discrimination Act (1992). Still, despite the major advances, debates in Australia and elsewhere on the nature of citizenship, constitutional development, and the future political status of disabled people seem to have been largely ignored to a point at which Meekosha (1999) has claimed that some 18% of the population who are the Australians with disabilities and handicaps have been excluded from protection under the law.

There are, as Meekosha (1999) has pointed out, several international conventions that together provide the foundation for an international bill of rights. While only the Convention on the Rights of the Child specifically refers to the rights of children with disabilities, there seems little doubt that these other conventions include people with disabilities. Key conventions include the International Covenant on Civil and Political Rights (1966); International Covenant on Economic, Social and Cultural Rights (1996/1976); International Convention on the Elimination of all forms of Racial Discrimination (1965); International Convention on the Elimination of all forms of Discrimination against Women (1979); Convention against Torture (1984); and the Convention on the Rights of the Child (1989).

Any existing doubt on the part of United Nations signatories about the application of these conventions to people with disabilities was vitiated by the World Conference on Human Rights in 1993. Paragraph 63 of the Vienna Declaration and Program states:

> The World Conference on Human Rights reaffirms that all human rights and fundamental freedoms are universal and thus unreservedly include persons with disabilities. Every person is born equal and has the same rights to life and welfare, education and work, living independently and active participation in all aspects of society. Any direct discrimination or other negative discriminatory treatment of a disabled person is therefore a violation of his or her rights. The World Conference on Human Rights calls on Governments, where necessary, to adopt or adjust legislation to assure access to these and other rights for disabled persons. (Darrow, 1996, p. 72)

A Philosophical Base

In virtually all societies, certain characteristics or attributes of people appear to be highly valued, while others are very much devalued. In Western society, for example, positively valued characteristics include wealth, youth, beauty, intelligence, and independence. People who do not always possess these attributes, for example, the poor, people with disabilities, the aged, are often devalued and consequently seen as having little or no social worth. These factors have resulted over a lengthy period from an ethic based upon perceptions of their social worth.

Devalued people are usually treated badly by society. Rejection is common and this poor treatment diminishes their dignity, growth, competence, and general well-being. It is evident to many who evaluate, for example, nursing homes and community boarding houses, that service managers, the public, and even the relatives of the person under management may be inappropriately pessimistic about the "client's" inability to respond positively and constructively to appropriate care regimes. However, being widely seen as filling a valued social role may help reduce or prevent a person from becoming devalued on the basis of some attribute or characteristic he or she possesses.

A social role can be described as a socially expected pattern of behavior that is usually assigned to, or assumed by an individual and which partially reflects the person's status in society. Examples of social roles are husband, sister, uncle, friend, neighbor, shopper, club member, churchgoer, worker, and volunteer.

The most recent definition of the term Social Role Valorization (SRV) is "the enablement, establishment, enhancement, maintenance and/or defence of valued social roles for people, particularly for those at value-risk—by using, as much as possible, culturally valued means" (Wolfensberger, 1992, p. 32). The term was developed to support the belief that the most explicit and ultimate goal of human services must be the creation, support, and defense of valued social roles for people who are at risk of social devaluation. The basic premise of SRV is that if a person's social role is generally valued by society, then other desirable things will be accorded to that person almost automatically, at least within the resources and norms of his or her society.

Wolfensberger and Thomas (1998) have contended that there are at least two ways of attaining valued social roles and life conditions for people at risk of devaluation. First, by the enhancement of people's *social image* or perceived value in the eyes of others, and second by enhancement of their *personal competence.* In his development of the SRV theory, Wolfensberger (1992) identified a number of elements that influence the social image attached to devalued people and the extent to which devalued people have opportunities to develop personal competence. For example, the physical settings where people live or work convey certain impressions and images depending on how aesthetically pleasing and comparable they are to physical settings used by valued people. As well, people can be either assisted or hindered in developing personal competence by the particular characteristics of the physical setting. Thus, a person who lives in a segregated setting with no accessible transport may have difficulty in developing skills in accessing the community.

In addition to the importance of the physical setting to a person's or group's enhancement of their social image and personal competencies, Wolfensberger (1983) highlights a number of other critically important elements. "Relationships and groupings" and "activities, programs and other uses of time" feature in both enhancement goals, and in the case of social image, "language and other forms of symbol and image" is very powerful.

Integration or inclusion in society, as opposed to segregation is an essential part of social role valorization. They refer to an ethic that underlies those measures and practices that maximize an individual's maximum participation in the cultural mainstream.

The philosophical acceptance by the international community of the existence of human rights and the intent that these should also refer to people with disabilities has been acknowledged by many societies through the legislative activities of their governments. The intent of these parliaments has been to enact legislation that seeks to ensure that the rights, generally spelled out in the preface to each Act, are honored in their implementation. Industry throughout the western or industrialized world is engaging in a gradual movement toward quality by the adoption, over time, of quality assurance standards. Regarding service provision to individuals with disabilities, it is hoped that service system quality assurance standards are being developed based on a clear deontological ethic based on an acceptance of general and specific rights.

Service Provision

The essence of service provision to people with disabilities is model coherency (Wolfensberger, 1975). The issue is concerned with whether or not a number of key variables combine to meet the specific needs of each client at a particular time in his or her life. Another way of understanding the fundamental service provision issue is to ask of the service system: Is this a system in which the right people are working with the right clients, who are properly grouped, doing the right things, using the right methods and consistently so?

CONCLUSIONS

The variables to be considered in studying the deontological ethics of service provision as it affects people with disabilities are related to client characteristics, which in turn devolve to client grouping by factors that enhance social and cultural value and client grouping by age-appropriateness. These factors together with an examination of the human management model in use, its program content and the processes through which content is delivered will, as a cluster, provide information on the ethical intent of those providing the service.

In Australia, the right to an array of comprehensive, coordinated, community-based services and supports has already given rise to the creation of service provision standards in the provision of vocational training to people with disabilities (Annison, Jenkinson, Sparrow, & Bethune, 1995). This needs to be widespread. If human service professionals are to practice successfully and competently, it seems essential that they cultivate a sound ethic that is closely related to the philosophical, social, and legislative frameworks that underpin service provision in contemporary national contexts.

REFERENCES

Annison, J., Jenkinson, J., Sparrow, W., & Bethune, E. (1995). *Disability: A guide for health professionals.* Melbourne: Thomas Nelson.

Cibinel, A., & Kiwanuka, J. (1998). *Human rights and disabled people.* Paper presented at UN Human Rights Vienna Conference, June 1998.

Cocks, E., & Stehlik, D. (1995). History of services. In J. Annison, J. Jenkinson, W. Sparrow, & E. Bethune (Eds.), *Disability: A guide for health professionals* (pp. 8–30). Melbourne: Thomas Nelson.

Conway, R., Bergin, L., & Thornton, K. (1996). *Abuse and adults with intellectual disability living in residential services.* Mawson, National Council on Intellectual Disability.

Darrow, M. (1996). International Human Rights Law and Disability: Time for an International Convention on the Human Rights of People with Disabilities. *Australian Journal of Human Rights, 3*(1), 69–96.

Fletcher, A. (1995). *Information kit on the United Nations Standard Rules for the Equalisation of Opportunities for Persons with Disabilities.* London: Disability Awareness in Action.

Fulcher, G. (1989). *Disabling policies? A comparative approach to education policy and disability.* London: The Falmer Press.

Gooding, C. (1994). *Disabling laws. Enabling acts: Disability rights in Britain and America.* London: Pluto Books.

Kelley, P., & Gale, G. (1998). *Towards excellence: Effective education for students with vision impairments.* North Rocks, NSW: North Rocks Press.

Meekosha, A. (1999). *Disability and human rights. Attorney General's Forum on Domestic Human Rights.* Canberra, ACT: Office of the Attorney General.

NSW Office of Disability. (1994). *Disability Services Act 1993 Statement of Principles.* Sydney: Government of New South Wales. Social Policy Directorate.

Sage, D. D., & Burrello, L. C. (1994). *Leadership in educational reform.* Sydney: Paul Brookes.

Wolfensberger, W. (1975). *Program Analysis of Service Systems* (3rd ed.). Toronto: National Institute on Mental Retardation.

Wolfensberger, W. (1983). *Guidelines for evaluators during a PASS, PASSING, or similar assessment of human service quality.* Downsview, ON: National Institute on Mental Retardation.

Wolfensberger, W. (1992). *A brief introduction to social role valorisation as a high order concept for structuring human services.* Syracuse, NY: Syracuse University Press.

Wolfensberger, W., & Thomas, S. (1998). Review of A. L. Chappell's (1992). Towards a sociological critique of the normalization principle. *International Social Role Valorization Journal, 2*(2), 12–21.

1

INTRODUCTION AND OVERVIEW

ROD G. BEATTIE

AUTHOR INTRODUCTION

In 1978 I started teaching at the Preschool for Hearing-Impaired Children at Brunskill School in Saskatoon, Saskatchewan, Canada. Twenty-two years ago—hard to believe, and yet it makes me one of the "novices" when I think of the people who are contributing chapters to this book. Sometimes I think my head is full—a personal learning limitation. I see the capacity of others as better—imagine the amount of information that they have taken in, integrated, and stored over their long careers in deafness, education, and psychology. They have so much to share.

My background involves degrees in psychology, special education, educational audiology, then more special education, and finally postdoctoral research experience in pragmatic language competencies of people with hearing impairments. With the exception of the psychology program when I started university—language, deafness, and teaching became common threads. These three areas are generally overlayed on my work experience as well. Besides the previously mentioned preschool teaching days, consulting and itinerant teaching in oral education settings are employment history features. Since 1985 I have also been involved in teacher training—first in Edmonton, at the University of Alberta and now for four years here in Sydney, Australia, at Renwick College. The courses I teach and supervise focus on language, speech, and auditory-oral/auditory-verbal methods. My sign language skills, unfortunately, are minimal having only taken introductory courses in American Sign Language and Auslan. I wish they were better. My deaf educational motto, if I have one, is "Try and 'figure out' what will be best."

A FEW QUOTES TO CONSIDER

From the ancient philosophers to modern day chairpersons of bankers associations ethics has, and remains, a much-discussed topic. Pondering thoughtfully on history, the writers of the online *Encyclopedia Britannica* suggested that,

> It is clear that ethics can only have come into existence when human beings started to reflect on the best way to live. This reflective stage emerged long after human societies had developed some kind of morality, usually in the form of customary standards of right and wrong conduct. The process of reflection tended to arise from such customs, even if in the end it may have found them wanting. Accordingly, ethics began with the introduction of the first moral codes. (*Encyclopedia Britannica,* 2000)

How these moral codes arose and the means of recording them is a life-study that tracks through diverse history, myth, and perhaps even magic.[1] Although there may be no agreement on what is ethical in some instances, there is thankfully concordance on, at least, a definition. The Concise Oxford defined ethics as 1: the science of morals in human conduct, 2a: moral principles, rules of conduct, 2b: a set of these (medical ethics). Merriam-Webster's listed 1: the discipline dealing with what is good and bad and with moral duty and obligation, 2a: a set of moral principles or values, 2b: a theory or system or moral values, 3: the principles of conduct governing an individual or group, 4: a guiding philosophy.

Highly similar definitions aside, the crux we may be most interested in is reflected in the following quotes. Spinrad and Spinrad (1979) expanded their probably borrowed dictionary definition by adding that ethics is "whatever society decides is the right way" (p. 88). Point taken. And recently, Frank Cicutto, chairman of the Australian Bankers Association, said, "You can have volumes of books and days of learned discussion on the subject of ethics and still end up with the question of, 'What is the right thing to do?'" (*Sydney Morning Herald,* February 12, 2000, p. 39).

Yes, what is the right thing to do?

IMPORTANCE OF THIS TOPIC

Ethics in Special Education has been an important recognized topic for many years. Reynolds and Fletcher-Janzen (1990) in their *Concise Encyclopedia of Special Education* summarized the key elements:

> Special education professionals are responsible for knowing the ethical standards of the profession and must be knowledgeable about the rights of exceptional children and their parents. Parents of special education children need to be informed of these rights, including the granting of consent for evaluation, diagnosis, and education. The right to privacy of the individual youngster and the family must be protected and all records and pertinent information kept confidential. When delivering an intervention, special education professionals are mainly responsible for choosing an educational alternative that would not be harmful, physically or mentally, to the handicapped youngster. (p. 413–414)

From this starting point the importance of ethics and a need for an extended discussion has surely grown for the early management and education of young children with hearing losses. A straw poll of professionals would likely support a motion that contends that a formal discussion is long past due. In the past, options for very young children with hearing losses, their parents and professionals, were fewer, more restricted, or perhaps even nonexistent. Canvassing the memories of senior citizens—even in developed countries—will find them recalling the "arrival" of the first wearable hearing aids. Similarly, these senior citizens will likely remember from the past that the choice of an educational program for a child with a significant hearing loss was au fait accompli. There was a "choice" of one—a school for the deaf, and perhaps even then that school was "a long way from home."

Now, the majority of the parents of deaf children in developed countries appear to have many more difficult decisions to make. (One might wonder if a parent's restricted choice made life easier in the past.) Presently, the scope of assistive listening equipment is huge and continuing to change and develop rapidly. Educational options may now span the service range from residential schools to full integration. Further, by combining these realities and today's varied language and methods of instruction, the parental decision-making role is even more complicated. Choices that span auditory/verbal to bilingual/bicultural: From one or more auditory/oral languages of the hearing majority to the natural visual/manual languages of the local Deaf community. Yes, many choices.

Technological development has certainly spurred many decisions with ethical implications. (Other contributing authors will develop this theme.) But briefly, there are also implications arising from an increased range of assessments for identifying the presence and degree of hearing loss at a very early age. These assessments can and will be more broadly and frequently applied. Highly accurate universal neonatal screening for a hearing loss is not a pipe dream in developed countries. Political will, once convinced of the cost benefits, will make it so, and then the children identified will refocus the ethical questions once again. The questions concerning assisted listening with its many options: Parents will need to make choices. The questions about language, learning/teaching methods, early childhood educational placements—again parents will be forced to make choices. Unlike parents from even just 20 years ago, they will have to make these decisions earlier, perhaps at a time when they are more "deaf naïve" than their forerunners.

Research, and the knowledge that comes from it is another factor that presses the development of questions and decisions about making ethical decisions. The neurological research that suggests or demonstrates that auditory deprivation results in fewer important interconnections forming in the infant's brain is information that will "pressure" the need to make amplification or language decisions. In contrast, sometimes it is the research that says we do not know the outcomes, like that relating to literacy development in children in bilingual/bicultural programs, that urges parents to make decisions with ethical riders.

Still, parents and professional must make decisions. Being a parent involves making choices and decisions whether one likes it or not. Sometimes it is of no consequence whether the ethical choices for these people arise from increased educational opportunity or variety, technological development and innovation, or basic growth, clarification, and/or questioning of knowledge. It would seem that the process has a pattern. An option, situation, or problem exists. The "involved" must research the opportunities and consequences to give direction to a situation or eliminate or minimize a problem. If possible, a mental balance sheet of positives and negatives may be developed with the gathering of the best available information. A hierarchy for the decision making is recognized. A prudent decision is made—perhaps with backup options formalized and coping-mechanisms considered—to support the decision through turbulent times or if a future reevaluation is necessary.

Beyond this introductory outline the importance of this topic of ethics and the education of young deaf children is simple: As involved professionals we have a duty to serve them well. Rightly or wrongly, criticism or blame has been often directed at medical or educational systems—especially those that drive it or provide support, and those that deliver the programs. If we are inadequate let us hope it because we are not yet sufficiently knowledgeable or lacking in resources (although still unacceptable). Let us hope that our inadequacies are not based in ignorance of or disregard to proper ethical procedures and standards.

To minimize our inadequacies in ethical areas perhaps we could, as a starting point, consider the Tri-Council (1996) suggestions, "good ethical reasoning, like good scientific reasoning, must be more than a matter of the mechanical and dogmatic application of rigid rules to fact situations. Ethical reasoning requires thought, insight, and sensitivity." (Tri-Council, 1996, p. 2–14).

MOTIVATION FOR UNDERTAKING THIS BOOK

The motivation for this book concerns the sincere desire to try to introduce and clarify the many ethical considerations concerning the provision of educational services and instruction for young children with hearing losses. The decisions that parents or guardians make on behalf of their children, often based on the contributions of educators, habilitation/rehabilitation specialists, medical personnel, and members of the Deaf community, deserve an airing in a formal fashion. Many of these decisions are very difficult, have long-lasting implications, and have "ethics" involvement. It is, perhaps, surprising that a book-length discussion of ethical issues in deafness has not been produced before.

The information on ethics in deaf education, in general, is limited. While the topic is a common discussion area for teachers of the deaf, few seem to know little about specific codes of ethics for their profession, or whether one even exists. Some teachers of the deaf may know, from contact with interpreters, that interpreters have a code of ethics for their work. (See for example National Association of the Deaf, 2000.) Other teachers, if active members of Auditory-Verbal International or the Council of Exceptional Children, will be aware that these groups have "codes of professional conduct." (See for example Estabrooks, 1994 & CEC Code of Ethics and Standards of Practice, 1997.) Tangentially, some deaf educators, from graduate work or research, will be familiar with ethics committees and their requirements. This last experience, however, will likely reflect the focus and guidelines used in the social sciences and humanities for research with human or animal studies. It will not consider the broader understanding of the ethical problems encountered by almost every parent of a child with a hearing loss or the professionals who work with them.

Developing this last thought, teachers and other front-line professionals soon realize that parents experience ethical issues as soon as they first lament unknowingly, or articulate formally, the question "Where do I go to get help?" At this point, it is quite possible that the professionals involved recognize the genesis of a host of ethical questions:

- Who should be providing the help?
- What are the issues concerning evaluation, assessment, amplification, implantation, visual communication systems, and sign languages?
- What technology route should the parents follow?
- What language should parents try to develop in their child?
- What educational settings and approach will best satisfy the needs of their child and parents for the present and foreseeable future?

Besides parents, involved professionals must also consider changes in the situation and deal with relevant ethical questions that concern such topics as "Where does my role or contribution end?" and "What happens if boundaries are overstepped?"

To date much of the information in the education of the deaf and ethical considerations has surfaced as a result of legal or quasi-legal interactions. (See for example Weisel's Chapter 6 for a discussion of this experience in Israel.) Often these debates and arguments are reflected in individual educational plans, assessment reports, and/or "rulings" on the choice of where a child will be educated. Those who have read ethics-related material will recognize that in special education legal actions and legislation feature prominently. Many will be familiar with references to the landmarks like *P.A.R.C. v. Commonwealth of Pennsylvania,* The Warnock Report, or Public Law 94–142. Broadly then, through these decisions, plans, reports, and legislative events we have taken "on board" more things ethical: What are the wishes and rights of the parent to make decisions on behalf of their children? What is the basis for discussions of the responsibilities of teachers to make sound decisions for the children under their care?

While these ethical questions are important, in the area of education of children with hearing losses they are only some of the "life" and educational decisions that are made for the child. In contrast, parents of a blind child will not likely ponder extensively the fundamental question, "What will be my child's first language? Or, How will they acquire that language?" Certainly, the parents of the deaf child have "extra-hard" decisions to make, and these decisions have complex flow-on implications. For example, if a hearing parent chooses a visual manual language for their child but fails to learn and use that language effectively themselves they or others may question their negligence. Or, by being made to feel guilty have they themselves been treated inappropriately? What recourse may the parent take if they feel an overly zealous individual or group has unduly influenced their decisions for their child with a hearing loss? How much persistence should there be in language learning using a particular methodology before a decision is made on the success or failure to acquire language using that method? And, if that language/method is considered a failure, what can be done about it and what changes should be made?

There are so many complex questions! The motivation for the book was simple.

INTENDED AUDIENCE

The intended or interested audience for a book of this nature is surely varied. I believe teachers, audiologists, speech-language pathologists, physicians, academics/researchers, advocates, and those in training to work in these professions will or should be interested. Having read the chapters ahead I have suggestions. Policy makers and researchers will do well to consider J. Schein's thoughts on demographics and deafness in Chapter 2. Parents, in particular, making decisions about life itself and lifestyle in general, for want of a better phrase, will find the focus of the third chapter by D. Power thought provoking. The discussion on defining disability and informed consent should have a wide appeal.

Parent and professionals alike will benefit from the material and examples in Chapter 4 where ethics and language choices are explored by D. Martin, M. Rodda, and S. Martin. E. Stewart and K. Ritter, in the Chapter 5, have explored the issues of contemporary assessment and hearing technology while introducing different ethical paradigms for decision making. For this chapter it would be easier to list those who would not be part of the interested audience. A. Weisel, in Chapter 6, and W. McCracken in 7 have both considered "things" educational—rights, options, placement, realities. Again parents and practicing teaching professionals, those intimately involved in working long-term with children with hearing losses and their families will form a nucleus of the intended audience. The Israeli and British experience should add a different dimension for readers in other locations.

The final focused chapters by G. Leigh and D. Stewart, may like J. Schein's chapter attract a particular audience: practicing teachers, academics/researchers, or teacher trainers. Leigh's Chapter 8, on curriculum considerations, from past experience will draw in questioning teachers and teachers-in-training, whereas Stewart's Chapter 9 on teacher training, will have a special appeal to both trainers and preservice professionals.

Parents and others may have particular interests—especially if they and their child/student/client are living the experience of a particular chapter's focus. There is no desire to limit anyone's interest. When outlining the concept of the book the original intended audience was smaller. I felt, however, the potential audience changed for several reasons as the work progressed. First, the audience grew because improved diagnosis and assessment techniques and new technical developments involved "other" nonspecialized professionals—computer analysis specialists, for example. Subsequently, the application of improved acoustic amplification or cochlear implants forces all concerned to change—to act quickly on first-language position for the child. Quite simply, many of the people listed in the "intended audience" will now be contributing earlier and more extensively to questions that impact on the "best interests" of the child—linguistically, educationally, culturally.

I also began to realize that the intended audience grew or changed as well from consumerism. Economic rationalization and other economic realities have spurred a different and demanding consumer. The media has effectively communicated much about medical and technological innovation. Many more parents are becoming knowledgeable consumers. It would be hard to imagine that there are many parents of a newly diagnosed deaf child who have not heard of a cochlear implant. Indeed, many parents with deaf children are soon aware of frontier research in areas such as hair-cell regeneration and gene therapy. Our "developed nations" status, with its rarefied media choices like the World Wide Web has played a huge role in educating people—albeit poorly at times. Via similar avenues, parents are also aware of having educational options for their child, and they are more willing to advocate and lobby to have their wishes and demands met than many in the past. Indeed, if modern parent-consumers feel they are not having their needs and desires met, the number who are willing to apply public/media pressure or pursue litigation has grown dramatically in many countries.

THE BOOK AHEAD

I believe the book ahead provides a great deal of thought-provoking information. Fighting a natural inclination to "streamline" I tried not to force the contributing authors into corners or boxes. I wanted their thoughts on the topic of ethics to emerge in a manner that reflects their thinking and their position. Still, I tried to use some structural devices outside and within their contributions like introductions, sample dilemmas, cases, and chapter addenda to support continuity. I hope the readers will appreciate these features.

Rationale for Design

Although the link between ethics and philosophical thought is strong, it was not the intention to dwell on philosophy—and certainly not to deliver an extended historical treatise on the development of ethics in philosophy. It is my hope that the book would have a "clarifying the current time" role and then, for those who are interested, that it stimulate the reader into deeper personal investigations through the follow-up references, suggestions, and ethical questions provided for further consideration.

I am sure the contributors to this book, hope, as do I, that the book represents a "developing" area for the education of the deaf. Ethical issues in the field of medicine and health receive considerable coverage. Human fertility, cloning, abortion, euthanasia, controversial medical treatment, and genetic manipulation represent but a brief list of topical issues. Presently, several items per week seem to make headlines in the national news. The one possible crossover area between the medical world and education of the deaf has been the ethical debate over the use of cochlear implants for children with severe and profound hearing losses. Still, the ethical debate on even this topic is limited. Indeed it is unfortunate that this debate is sometimes just a sermon preached to the converted, or a forum where propaganda is lobbed at the "enemy" from the tribal trenches.

Like the statement by the Tri-Council that focused on ethics in research, the rationale for the design of the book is to support the development of ethical thinking:

> The intention is to guide and evoke thoughtful actions rather than to generate formulae or algorithms for ethical decision-making. This is very much in keeping with the best uses of the four familiar principles [respect for persons, non-maleficence, beneficence, & justice] of health care ethics. (Tri-Council, 1996, p. 2–2)

The book ahead, as I envisioned it, is a beginning. I know of no other focused book that has combined the factors of ethics, education, and deafness to discuss a variety of topics that concern parents and professionals who have and continue to work with young children with hearing losses. I found I agreed with Newell's (1991) critical evaluation of a paper from the National Health and Medical Research Council that contends that the bioethics literature has been too dominated by medical discourse. Newell argued "that their paper has neglected to account for the social nature of disability and handicap" (p. 46). Although I was not driven completely by Newell's statement, I had similar feelings.

Personally, studying both general ethics in research documents and professional codes of ethical conduct has been valuable. I invite others to follow this avenue. These sources illustrated two things. First, they give labels for topics that need to be familiar to parents and teachers of children with hearing losses. Important topics like: Respect for Persons; Non-maleficence, Beneficence, Justice; Coherence, Prudence, and Pragmatism; Responsibility as an Individual or Part of a Collective; Free and Informed Consent, Harms and Benefits; Privacy and Confidentiality; and Exploitation. Second, the codes made one think about the familiarity that an educator should have with their professional obligations. Still, the growth of information on ethics, deafness, and education is probably "too little— too slow." Few, I suspect, would argue against a broader ethical discussion.

Description of the Book

The approach that I have taken is to ask a cross section of very experienced people—academics, researchers, educators—to prepare concise readable chapters on assigned topics in the area of deafness, education, and ethics. The authors were instructed to consider that the material, although it may originate in the academic milieu, should also be suitable to those unfamiliar with the area, but keen to learn. I wanted material that new parents, mainstream educators, teachers of the deaf in training, and educator/administrators from general education, rehabilitation, and medicine could understand.

To introduce or support the chapters the authors were asked to include illustrative ethical dilemmas where possible. Besides provoking thoughts in the readers for the chapter's contents, I wanted these dilemmas to give a human quality or reference. In some chapters the authors choose to build their chapter around a single illustrative case study. Others used a series of different dilemmas. As a secondary aspect of the introduction to each chapter, I asked the authors to introduce themselves—a personal statement. In these statements I wanted them to describe their backgrounds, perspectives, biases or credos that they might have and hold. Some statements are short—others longer. Regardless, I believe they develop the author's personality and should increase the reader's interest in the topic.

To conclude each chapter the individual authors were asked to include three things:

1. A list of the important points from their chapter—either deduced or experienced.
2. A suggested list of relevant materials for follow-up by interested readers. And,
3. Present a list of ethical questions reflecting or extending the chapter's content.

For some of the authors, I assumed this task with ongoing communication. In some chapters the lists are quite extensive—in others they are brief. In all cases the lists should be thought as "works in progress", especially the list of resources and questions for consideration.

Arrangement of Chapters

The book consists of 10 chapters. The first and the last, I originally thought of as bookends. I hoped to outline in the first and summarize in the last. As the project evolved, I felt I needed to give a bit more design information in the first. For the final chapter the plans also changed. An extensive summary of my colleague's work seemed redundant. Like many things in writing and research, their questions spawned more questions and ideas. Thus, the last chapter is more about introducing some topics that deserved, at least, an initial airing.

The eight central chapters are also loosely "theme" organized. The first quartet focuses on the ethical areas and problems that concern the child with a hearing loss who is between birth and 3 years of age. Thus topics such as demographics, technology, first language, method of communication, and assessment and hearing intervention take center stage. The second quartet are more likely to consider the older child from 3 to 6 years of age. In these chapters the access to education programs, available options, curriculum considerations, and the training and competencies of teachers in formal educational programs for children with hearing losses are featured.

Although there has been a pronounced attempt to coordinate the material and chapters, I have always hoped that the reader would be able to recognize their particular area of interest and that each of the chapters would stand independently.

What Do the Contributing Authors Bring?

The answer to this question subheading is years and years of practical experience and research on a huge number of topics concerning deafness and deaf education. It would be difficult to imagine a topic in deaf education that one or more of the contributing authors have not directly experienced. From international/national investigations to case studies—the authors have researched and disseminated their results. The contributing author's published work has featured people who have triumphed and those who have struggled.

Among the authors there are individuals who know deafness or hearing loss intimately—with mild to profound losses, or through immediate family members. The connection to ethics for most, however, has not been the raison d'être for their involvement in deafness and deaf education. For some, interest in ethics grew out of observation and involvement. Parents have told of experiences they and their children have had. Teachers have lamented the difficulties they have experienced while teaching. Graduate teachers-in-training have posed ethical dilemmas: "What happens if…? What would you do when…? I feel incapable of coping because…" Research, too, has raised ethical issues for some.

Very few of the contributing authors are graduate-trained ethicists. Generally our training comes from education, speech pathology, audiology, psychology, child development. We do, however, care for this topic. Care pressing us to be concerned enough to make a start and perhaps lay some groundwork. I know I want those who are involved with young children with hearing impairments to think about the topic. To, perhaps, understand the issues and questions that are germane in topics like diagnosis, single versus multiple disabilities, family dynamics, language use, method of learning, assessment, appliances, instruction methods, educational placement, curriculum choices, teacher preparation. Certainly, not all of these topics represent ethical dilemmas for all children with hearing impairments and their parents, but all seem to have the potential to pose a dilemma.

Acknowledging Realities

The reality I was forced to acknowledge for this book was simply that I did not have a tried and tested model from which to start. I believe the book represents a new area for education of the deaf. Certainly there would be many more models to choose from if it was a book on ethics and human fertility, general disability, cloning, abortion, euthanasia, controversial medical treatment, or genetic manipulation. Yes, there is the crossover discussion of ethics and cochlear implantation, but as I suggested earlier, this too is limited.

In acknowledging realities I quickly realized that trying to keep a pragmatic attitude was one of the most difficult things to do. I, like everyone else, have my positions, opinions, and beliefs. I wished all three were based in knowledge and truth, but I recognize that this is not the case. It concerns me that my gut-instincts, emotional bias, and stubbornness may play a substantive role in my decision making. To counteract my concerns I have tried to keep reminding myself about maintaining a degree of neutrality and open-mindedness. I try to read material from the other side of the fence. To minimize the urge to trash or scream at "difficult" material, I have tried to focus on questions. Which position has the most questions? Which questions are the most difficult to answer or have the greatest amount of unknown? By thinking in this manner, I find that I am forced to acknowledge realities.

Title Terms and Other Definitions

This book contains an extended glossary in the reference section with terms and relevant phrases that arose during the production of this book. The glossary contents will not be duplicated here. Rather, for this heading, I would like to focus on the key elements from the working title of the book: ethics, deaf education, and the first 6 years.

The "ethics" element of the title, as I considered it, was concerned with "supporting or doing the right thing" or "making or contributing to the best decision" for a child with hearing loss and their parents or caregivers. The definition was not pushed to its limits. Neither were the words that philosophers have struggled with challenged to the end. Thinking pragmatically was the aim and an effort was made to remain true to that desire. I wanted to read the recorded thoughts of a range of experienced others who have considered and reflected on the topics of ethics and deafness. I hoped the material they would provide would be both a challenge to the "deaf familiar" and a benefit to the "deaf naïve."

The "deaf education" and "first 6 years" were essentially linked elements, albeit separated by a colon in the working title. The "education" component of deaf education for the purpose of this book should be thought of in the broad sense. Education is referring to the process of engendering or facilitating learning in children with hearing losses: learning that occurs through the interaction of development or maturation, parenting, and early child/adult interaction. It also includes learning that occurs for children with teachers in educational settings. This sweeping definition of education also recognizes the first processes are much more informal than the latter, especially when the parenting of the very young is taken into account. Thus, to restate, think broadly: Deaf education—the process of learning and education for all children with some degree of hearing impairment from birth to age 6.

The book does suggest a deaf education distinction between 0 to 3 and 4 to 6 in the arrangement of the chapters. I had, however, no intention of suggesting that a watershed exists in the informal and formal educational processes for all young children with a hearing loss. There was no intention of saying that "learning" through maturation, parenting, and early child/adult interaction is limited to the younger age. No intention, either, of saying that teachers take over at the 4- to 6-year age range with a suitcase of teaching techniques, curriculums, and educational materials. The two age grouping reflects a simple observed reality: parents spend more time "educating" the child when they are younger—and teachers play an increased role in when the children are older. Again, the aim was to think about "deaf education" and the "first 6 years" in a pragmatic way. Certainly links between parents and teachers exist throughout the age range, and the ultimate goals held by both are probably very similar. Both are likely hoping that the development and learning of the child with a hearing loss occurs in a fashion such that the child has the knowledge, skills, and abilities of other children of a similar chronological age.

The word "deaf" in deaf education is also meant to be thought of inclusively, but still highlights three more definitions: hard of hearing, deaf, and Deaf. Hard of hearing refers to those children "whose hearing, though impaired, is used as a primary modality for auditory speech perception and language acquisition" (Morris, 1992, p. 91). Deaf, spelled with a lowercase "d" is the audiological grouping of children with hearing losses. The "deaf" then are those "unable to usefully perceive sounds in the environment with or without the use of a hearing aid" and perhaps "unable to use hearing as the primary way to gain information" (Smith, Luckasson, & Crealock, 1995, p. 424). Deaf with an uppercase "D" refers to those with a cultural-linguistic affiliation to a community of similar others.

Now taking the words "deaf education" together, and referring to the more formal educational approaches that involve teachers, the two words encompass for this book, as Morris (1992) states, the "three main educational approaches to help the child who has a hearing loss" (p. 69). The *Oral* approach where the focus is on using listening and spoken communication "so that they can become part of mainstream society" (Smith et al., 1995, p. 452). (With acknowledgment to the possible variations like (a) the auditory-verbal, unisensory, acoupedic programs where visual stimuli is minimized, and (b) the multisensory approach were more visual stimuli like natural gesture, lipreading, and/or fingerspelling may be used.) The *Total Communication* approach where Turkington and Sussman (1992) state that "rather than focus on one specific training method, parents and teachers … try to decide which mode is best for a child in any one situation. Options can include speechreading, speech, sign language, auditory training and amplification, writing, audiovisual methods, fingerspelling and graphics" (p. 187). And finally the *Manual* approach, where sign language is the primary means of instruction, and now includes the Bilingual-Bicultural methods where a natural sign language is developed as a first language, and then subsequently used to develop at least literacy in the oral language of the larger hearing community/culture.

INTREPIDLY LOOKING AHEAD

I have struggled with what I might call this last section. The current heading must do because I believe the readers should approach the chapters fearlessly. We had to. Certainly, each author accepted the challenge when I approached them to contribute to the book. I am quite sure that I might receive a different response if I asked them now. I was not surprised that a common phrase in their correspondence during the writing process was, "This has been much more difficult than I thought it would be." I found it so myself. I could quickly write my personal thoughts on topic X or topic Y, but when my academic insecurities surfaced and I found myself wanting to quote or reference—the appropriate or apt citation was often unavailable or did not exist. Oh for the want of a *Book of Shadows.*

Since wishes aren't horses that beggars might ride, neither may I nor the contributing authors be all things to all people. Backgrounds, knowledge, experiences, and beliefs have colored our perspective on the ethical issues identified and addressed, purposely excluded, and unconsciously forgot in each chapter. Constraints of time and space may have limited some topics. For others, the selected topics within their chapter may have been a conscious choice either because they were "easy" and they felt confident they could undertake them or perhaps a topic was avoided because they felt they could not do justice to it. It is also quite likely that not everyone sees the same ethical problems and possible dilemmas as others do in this complex area. I will say that I have become acutely aware that one person's passionate problem can be another's passing piffle. In saying this I believe even this information is important. So if a statement or omission sparks a challenge, then well and good. Take up the pen and nail the challenge to a public wall so that others can read it.

Trying to Identify the Key Questions

In this huge topic of ethics I have struggled to keep things simple. Although taken out of context from J. D. Mabbott's book, *An Introduction to Ethics,* I loved the statement, "The key words in morals are 'good,' 'right,' and 'ought.'" And the linkage of these words is to "duty." Although sometimes lost in a whirl of philosophical circle language, this simple sentence made sense. No matter whether the chapters concerned demographics, first language, communication, or any of the other topics, I found it helpful to keep these four words in mind. Each of Mabbott's key words can be used effectively for different topics of interest: Is the choice of a particular language a *good* one for a specific child? Have we made the *right* educational program decision for a child and the child's family? Is there something we *ought* to do to inform the parents of the consequences of making a certain decision or choice of assistive listening equipment? To be sure, it is not difficult to link these questions to duty in short order. I would not like to leave the impression that there are simple answers. Indeed I know that is not the case, but I do believe that the link is easy to make.

Identifying the Players and Their Positions

As I searched and read material dealing with or commenting on ethics and moral issues, I was surprised at how few people state their personal position directly. I wonder should this not be a priority? Lynas (1999), in discussing selection of communication approach, said "the most important factor, in my view, is which of the alternative options available to the young child will be least constraining and will leave most options open to the deaf child on becoming an adult" (p. 124). Although "in my view" was not highlighted, at least it was stated. The reader is not left wondering. Personally I like this.

REFERENCES

American Speech-Language-Hearing Association. (1995). Code of Ethics of the American Speech-Language-Hearing Association. In F. H. Silverman, *Speech, language, and hearing disorders* (pp. 228–232). Needham Heights, MA: Allyn & Schuster.

Balkany, T., Hodges, A. V., & Luntz, M. (1996). Update on cochlear implantation. *Otolaryngol-Clin-North America, 29*(2), 277–289.

Council for Exceptional Children (CEC). (1997). *Code of ethics and standards of practice* [On-line]. Available: http://www.cec.sped.org/ps/code.htm.

Encyclopedia Britannica. (2000). *Ethics* [On-line]. Available: http://www.britannica.com.

Encyclopedia Britannica. (2000). *Human rights* [On-line]. Available: http://www.britannica.com.

Estabrooks, W. (Ed.). (1994). *Auditory-verbal therapy for parents and professionals.* Washington, DC: Alexander Graham Bell Association for the Deaf.

Lynas, W. (1999). Communication options. In J. Stokes (Ed.). *Hearing impaired infants: Support in the first eighteen months* (pp. 98–128). London: Whurr.

Mabbott, J. D. (1966). *An introduction to ethics.* London: Hutchinson.

Merriam-Webster's collegiate dictionary (10th ed.). (1999). Springfield, MA: Merriam-Webster.

Morris, D. W. H. (1992). *Dictionary of communication disorders* (2nd ed.). London: Whurr.

National Association of the Deaf. (2000). *NAD interpreter code of ethics* [On-line]. Available: http://nad.policy.net/proactive/newsroom/release.vtml?id=17200.

Newell, C. (1991). A critical evaluation of the NH & MRC's "The Ethics of Limiting Life—Sustaining Treatment" and related perspectives on the bioethics of disability. *Australian Disability Review, 4,* 46–57.

Reynolds, C. R., & Fletcher-Janzen, E. (Eds.). (1990). *Concise encyclopedia of special education.* New York: John Wiley & Sons.

Smith, D. D., Luckasson, R., & Crealock, C. (1995). *Introduction to special education in Canada: Teaching in an age of challenge.* Scarborough, ON: Allyn & Bacon.

Spinrad, L., & Spinrad, T. (1979). *Speaker's lifetime library.* Englewood Cliffs, NJ: Prentice-Hall.

Sydney Morning Herald. (2000, February 12). Frank Cicutto Interview. *Sydney Morning Herald,* p. 39.

The Concise Oxford Dictionary (8th ed.). (1991) Oxford: Clarendon.

Tri-Council Working Group. (1996). *Code of conduct for research involving humans.* Ottawa, ON: Minister of Supply and Services.

Turkington, C., & Sussman, A. E. (1992). *The encyclopedia of deafness and hearing disorders.* New York: Facts On File.

APPENDIX

Important or Main Points

- For the purpose of this book the ethical issues concerning deafness and education were "compartmentalized" by age. This is an artificial division and indeed there are ethical issues that span both age ranges.
- Following a discussion of the importance, motivation, and structural features of the book, there was a discussion of trying to identify key questions and players. First language, modality, and access were all identified as central to both questions and players. Many issues seem easier to relate to in the question format: Is a mother tongue or first language (a) the language that your parents speak, or (b) a language that is most accessible through the available distance sense organs?
- The suggestion is made that technology development is charging many areas of the topic of ethics and deafness.

Follow-up References or Suggestions

- For an introduction to ethics several "older" books serve an interested reader well. Mabbott, J. D. (1996). *An introduction to ethics.* London: Hutchinson, and, Williams, B. (1993). *Morality: An introduction to ethics* (reissued ed.). Cambridge: Cambridge University Press, are two suggestions.
- A useful introduction to bioethics is Shannon, T. A., (1997). *An introduction to bioethics* (3rd ed.). Mahwah, NJ: Paulist Press.
- There are also a large number of sources available on the Internet. Quality of the material should be questioned in some instances, but many sources provide an excellent introduction. A starting point suggestion would be: Encyclopedia Britannica. (2000). [On-line]. Available: http://www.britannica.com. A simple search using terms such as "ethics" or "human rights" will provide the reader with a collection of material.

Ethical Questions for Consideration

- Is the topic of ethics, deafness, and education worthy of an extended treatment from the educational perspective or can it be adequately covered by fields like health-science and psychology?
- Is it possible to identify which scenario is more realistic for a given family: Using a combination of technology and educational activities so that the child learns the oral language of home and community, versus teaching the parents and the deaf child a visual language so that the child may develop that language in a natural manner?
- Is it possible at this time to overcome a hearing loss with technology designed to allow the child to naturally access the oral language of his or her

parents, family, and their community? If not now, is this "technological solu-tion" a possibility in the near future?

- Is it possible, without disenfranchisement, to compliment or supplement non-signing parents with others who can communicate effectively with the deaf child to allow the child to naturally access a visual language? Do we know what this might mean for the parent-child relationship?

NOTES

[1] Consider King Arthur and his Round Table knights an an example of the possible influence of myth and magic on ethical thinking. For now, however, I'll leave this point for others.

PART

I

FROM BIRTH TO
THREE YEARS

The following four chapters focus on ethical areas and problems that generally concern parents and professionals who have, or work with, children with a hearing losses between birth and three years of age. Topics include demographics, development of technology and science, conceptualization of disability, informed choice, first language, method of communication, assessment, and choice of hearing equipment. Often the questions that arise during this time play a role in all subsequent ethical dilemmas and decisions. If, for example, a first-language decision is made at 14 months of age when the child's deafness is confirmed, it is not as if everyone can start afresh four years later because the limitations of the decision for this child are now clear. As much as we might sometimes wish, wiping the slate clean is not an option.

Although there was a basic framework provided for the authors at the beginning and a concerted effort to coordinate the chapters as they were written, there are chapter variations, as one might expect. The substantial variation of national perspective and experience is central to many differences, but then so is the nature of being an academic or practitioner from different disciplines. Thus, both the book's design and the authors' products evolved. I have always felt that many readers would know their particular areas of interest and because of that I hoped that each of the chapters would stand independently to meet these interests. Although I feel this has been achieved, there is a linkage and in some instances some overlap of the topics. I do not see the overlap as negative; the perspective is different, and this difference can be enlightening.

In the second chapter—the first of the quartet—J. Schein discusses the broader issues of deafness and ethics with an overview of demographics. He opens with the question, "What can be unethical about the demography of deafness?" Using the question and a borrowed anecdote, a series of issues are drawn out for the consideration of the readers. The cliché "more to this than meets the eye" is apt. Wisdom from experience, problems with definitions, the effects of time and geography are all part of the discussion. Perhaps more than in other chapters Schein is able to discuss options for moving toward problem minimization.

In the third chapter D. Power takes us into the area of conceptualization of disability and in ethical dilemmas arising from the march of science and technological change. The perspective, however, is not exclusively focused on hearing aid and cochlear implants and similar widgit development and refinement. Rather, Power's "technology" focus starts with life itself. Technology, in the broad sense—through genetic screening and genetic engineering—may soon allow us to "know the outcome" of a pregnancy, leaving us with the ethical dilemma of what to do next. Options such as "correction" or "curing" and "termination" are discussed. Extending his exploration, Power introduces discussions on defining disability, informed consent, and the reaction of others to "reasonable medical treatment" that may or may not be followed.

The fourth chapter by D. M. Martins, M. Rodda, and S. Martins explores the topic of language and mode of communication for the child with a hearing loss and the family. A particular focus concerns first language for the child and the ethical dilemmas concerning choice and outcomes for making that choice. An introduction and historical perspective on language opens the chapter. This is followed by an overview of language and communication. The ethical dimensions of language choice is discussed in the body of the text with the "assistance" of several illustrative cases that highlight a variety of first language conditions, possibilities, and questions. Perhaps the key question highlighted in the "reflections" section deserves the longest ponder by all readers: "How many professionals have a perspective of the whole life span of our students and clients?"

The last of the first four chapters concerns ethics of assessment in general and then follow-through for the tough question of whether to proceed with implantation for the child who may be a candidate for this technology. E. Stewart and K. Ritter provide an extended narrative as a basis for their discussion. They then apply principlism, the most applied approach in bioethics, to consider the issues raised in the extended narrative. Some might believe that twists and turns were introduced in the narrative to complicate the picture, but those with experience will recognize that this would not be necessary. Each life-story of every family has these complexities—contrived events, as might be found in fiction, are not needed. Even the simplest life is easily complicated with small events.

Enjoy the journey ahead—I know I have.

2

ETHICAL CONSIDERATIONS IN THE DEMOGRAPHY OF DEAFNESS

JEROME D. SCHEIN

AUTHOR INTRODUCTION

The demography of deafness has intrigued me for four decades. The notion of counting needles in a haystack appealed to me from the start. However, I had no academic preparation for the task: a doctorate in Clinical Psychology hardly qualifies one to undertake the overlapping specialties of demography, psychology, and sociology. So I have had to learn "on the job." In that respect, I have had the gracious assistance of so many experts, both in demography and deafness, that space will not permit my listing them all. Suffice it to say that without their support I could not have succeeded in completing 30-some studies, including the National Census of the (U.S.) Deaf Population and Canadians with Impaired Hearing.

The most dangerous pitfall in assuming the pose of an expert on deaf populations' sizes and characteristics is THE EASY ANSWER. Once you are marked as having gathered some data, you can expect questions that can only receive qualified answers—ethically. Most questioners do not want qualified answers: "Just give me the numbers, professor, not a lecture." Withstanding such assaults takes a large dose of humility and a willingness to protect your integrity against humoring others. In what follows, I hope that I have been true to both antidotes to "giving easy answers." Why that sick approach should be avoided is the burden of the article that follows.

A CASE TO CONSIDER

What can be unethical about the demography of deafness? Asked another way, What have ethics to do with determining the size and characteristics of a deaf population? This chapter addresses these questions, while providing concepts relevant to studying aggregates of deaf people.

A colleague writes (and I quote with editing to protect confidentiality and broaden the generality of the anecdote):

> A few years ago I was invited to two different legislative committees on the same day. The Educational Committee discussed sign language interpreting on television. The legislators asked me how many deaf people would benefit from such a service. The deaf people who attended the meeting wanted me to give as large a number as possible since that would make the service more reasonable. An hour later I participated in a meeting of the Welfare Committee, which was considering tax exemptions for deaf people. This time the deaf participants wanted me to give as small a number as possible, since a large number would make the cost seem too large. Trying to be as honest as possible, and given the fact that I don't have really accurate data, I chose to explain how I arrived at my estimates. I thought that if the legislators got the impression that I'm playing with the numbers in order to improve the chances of the legislation passing they would either disregard my testimony or would not invite me again as an expert, or both. So I presented my best and honest estimates. As a result: (a) deaf people were dissatisfied with my presentations; (b) I'm no longer invited for this purpose; (c) both bills passed. I concluded that political decisions are not much influenced by facts and academicians—especially the honest ones—are, and perhaps should be, isolated individuals.

My colleague's dilemma is one I have also faced. The one question that has been asked of me most frequently in my 40 years of association with deafness research is "How many deaf people are there?" Sometimes the question is as broad as that. Other times it is asked about deafness in a specific geographical location or about a segment of the deaf population. In every instance, the questioner assumes that there is a ready answer, either in numbers or rates. Such naiveté makes it difficult to give an ethical response.

ETHICS DEFINED

For me, ethics refers to a code of professional conduct, one that identifies moral principles that guide a profession or professional activity. The code specifies the right and wrong ways to conduct professional business. It represents a consensus among those practicing the profession and the public. Demographers of deafness are a tiny group without their own professional organization, so no published ethical code exists. Each demographer abides by the ethics of whatever profession to which she or he belongs. Given that circumstance, I offer a single moral principle: *be honest.* It is a principle easy to state, but often difficult to follow.

A magazine devoted to deaf affairs advertises that the number of deaf people in the United States numbers 20,000,000—an astonishingly large number. The magazine does not bother to define deafness or to say from whence they derive this figure.[1] But since the publication's intended audience consists of *early deaf-ened* people, it must puzzle its readers, who expect a much larger number of persons like themselves than exists. Allowing readers to free associate as to the meaning of "deaf people" is deceptive. If such a statement were offered by a demographer, I would label it unethical.

Honesty sometimes begets annoyance, even occasional belligerence—at least in my experience. To give an honest answer to any of the questions, I usually must inquire in return as to what the questioner means. This generates reactions like "All I want is the number, not a lecture." Or, "You professors can't say what time it is without explaining how watches are made." More emphatic rejoinders are not suitable for this chapter, so I leave it to the reader to consider what they may be like.

Why the hostility to ethical answers? Why should it be so difficult to answer the how-many questions? First, because defining terms can be laborious. Second, the deaf population is a moving target, one that not only varies over time, but from place to place. To avoid giving misleading estimates, one must constantly update them or else indicate that they are based on earlier efforts that may no longer be accurate.

DEFINITIONS OF DEAFNESS

An honest answer specifies its parameters. Foremost among these is the definition of deafness. To illustrate the problem, I hark back to my first efforts to answer that question for myself. I consulted several monographs then considered authoritative. Each provided a different estimate of the size of the United States deaf population, ranging from 120,000[2] to 15,000,000.[3] Such enormous discrepancies were disconcerting, until I realized that each author defined "deafness" differently.

That experience prompted me to delve into the variety of definitions of deafness—a quest that may seem academic, a professorial exercise, but one that also involves ethics.[4] To give an honest answer, one must first be sure that it fits the question. To do so requires asking the questioners what they mean. And that prompts the reactions of annoyance, since most people have not thought about the numerous ways "deafness" is construed. I am asserting that it is unethical to assume a questioner's meaning. At the least, the ethical answer must make clear that more than one answer is correct, depending on the definition chosen, and alert the questioner that the reply being given would differ if based on other factors.

TIME

The size of the deaf population varies over time. It changes as deaf babies are born and deaf people die—as they immigrate and emigrate into and out of particular areas. Because most populations change over time, questions are usually concerned with the *relative* size of the deaf population (i.e., what proportion of a general population is deaf?). The answer must deal with two estimates—the sizes of the general and of the deaf populations. Both change over time, which means that ethical answers will have to be carefully couched in terms that indicate the tentative nature of the answer. For example, the size of the U.S. population, determined by the Bureau of the Census every 10 years at a cost of billions of dollars, is, it is hoped, accurate within 5%. So its present size may actually lie between 266,000,000 and 294,000,000. For a rare condition like prelingual deafness, the difference between the two denominators will greatly influence the rate, even if the numerator is absolutely accurate.

Are changes in the estimated size of the deaf population really so dramatic that one must be cautious in defining the specific era? Consider one of many possible examples. Table 2.1 presents the number of deaf people in the United States as determined by the U.S. Bureau of the Census between 1830 (the first census) and 1930. Why stop at 1930? Because the Bureau did not gather this statistic after 1930. The explanation for having stopped counting deaf persons is worth quoting:

> No high degree of accuracy is to be expected in a census of the blind and of deaf-mutes
> carried out by the methods which it has been necessary to use thus far in the United States…[5]

Note that what the Bureau regarded as inaccuracies resulted from "the methods" then used. As discussed below, newer methods have enabled demographers to achieve more reliable results. Clearly, however, the possibility remains that the rates obtained by the Bureau, though fluctuating widely, did reflect the true proportion of the population that was deaf *at each time*. The Bureau's distress over

TABLE 2.1   Prevalence and Prevalence Rates per 100,000 Population of Deaf-Mutes.[a] United States, 1830–1930

Year	Number	Rate/100,000
1930	57,084	46.5
1920	44,885	42.5
1910	44,708	48.6
1900	24,369	32.1
1890	40,592	64.8
1880	33,878	67.5
1870	16,205	42.0
1860	12,821	40.8
1850	9,803	42.3
1840	7,678	45.0
1830	6,106	47.5

Source: U.S. Bureau of the Census. (1931). *The blind and deaf-mutes in the United States: 1930.* Washington, DC: United States Government Printing Office.

[a] The Bureau's term, which is now unacceptable, both socially and scientifically.

the wide swings in their estimates of the relative sizes of the deaf population—from 67.5, in 1880, to 32.1, in 1900—may reflect a belief that the proportion of deaf to the general population should be fairly constant. Such reasoning overlooks the effects of epidemics affecting newborns (such as the rubella epidemics of 1963–1965, in the United States) and bouts of meningitis attacking persons of all ages. These events can significantly increase the proportion of deaf persons in the general population. Differential birth and death rates are also important factors that must be considered. Whatever the case may be, time is a significant factor in estimating the size of the deaf population.

GEOGRAPHY

The incidence and prevalence rates[6] for deafness differ from country to country and within countries. Table 2.2 displays rates collected for an earlier study (Schein, 1973). Highest and lowest rates differ by almost nine times! Note also

TABLE 2.2   Prevalence Rates per 100,000 Population for Prelingual Deafness: Based on Censuses, 1930–1956

Country	Year	Rate/100,000
Peru	1940	300.0
Honduras	1935	137.9
Finland	1950	130.7
Japan	1947	118.0
Switzerland	1953	93.7
Sweden	1930	86.9
Iceland	1948	75.8
India	1931	66
Canada	1941	62.6
Egypt	1937	60
Belgium	1950	59.5
Norway	1930	53.0
Union of South Africa	1936	49.4
France	1946	47
United States	1930	46.5
Northern Ireland	1956	45.1
Denmark	1940	43.4
West Germany	1950	43.1
Mexico	1940	39.1
Australia	1933	35.1

Source: Schein, J. D. (1973). Hearing disorders. In L. T. Kurland, J. F. Kurtzke, & I. D. Goldberg, *Epidemiology of neurologic and sense organ disorders* (p. 276–304). Vital and Health Statistics Monographs, American Public Health Association. Cambridge: Harvard University Press.

the large discrepancies between neighboring countries—Finland (130.7), Sweden (86.9), Norway (53.0), Denmark (43.4). Contiguous countries such as Canada (62.6) and the United States (46.5) also had sizable differences in their rates for the years reported by their governments' respective statistical organizations.

Even within countries the prevalence rates can differ greatly. In Peru, the lowest rate per 100,000 for prelingual deafness[7] was found in the region encompassing the city of Callao (30), while the highest rate occurred in the mountainous province of Amazonas (843). The enormous difference is accountable by other than methodological reasons.[8] Unrecognized, the discrepancies in the relative rates for the two regions would lead to wasteful situations. If services had been provided on the basis of the national average rate of 300 per 100,000, it would have overestimated by 10 times the amount needed by Callao and underestimated Amazonas's needs by nearly 3 times.

An additional example of differences in prevalence rates between a country's geographic regions can be found in data for the United States (see Table 2.3). The proportion of the population that is deaf in the Northeast (173) contrasted markedly from that in the North Central region (242) and each region's prevalence rate differed from that of the entire country—cautioning against applying averages from large areas to their components.

OTHER FACTORS

For educators and rehabilitators, the age at onset[9] of the deafness is crucial in determining how to manage it. Persons deafened prelingually differ dramatically from those with the same degree of impairment suffered in late adulthood. The former will have great difficulty acquiring speech, whereas the latter will undoubtedly

TABLE 2.3   Prevalence Rates per 100,000 Population for Prevocational Deafness[a] by Census Regions, United States, 1971

Region[b]	Rate/100,000
United States	203
Northeast	173
North Central	242
South	196
West	194

Source: Schein, J. D., & Delk, M. T. (1974). *The deaf population of the United States.* Silver Spring, MD: National Association of the Deaf.

[a] Onset of deafness prior to 19 years of age.

[b] As defined by the U.S. Bureau of the Census. See source for states in each region.

retain it. The language development of the former will present problems, whereas the latter's will be largely unaffected by the loss of hearing. Persons prelingually deaf will most often become members of the Deaf community, but those deafened in adulthood seldom join it. So answering the question how many deaf people requires specification of when in the developmental cycle the deafness occurred.

Prevalence rates also differ by gender and economic status.[10] Although we will not illustrate them here, these are differences that can be significant. Understanding the factors that contribute to a group's size can have important implications for service providers. For example, because deafness occurs more frequently in males than females, when building a school for deaf students, more males than female-oriented facilities should be provided, based on the probable difference in the proportion of the two genders over time.

TOWARD SOLVING THE PROBLEMS

If the preceding discussion proves cogent, you should be convinced that there is no easy answer to the question how many deaf persons? Its answer must specify relevant factors: the degree of impairment, the age at onset, the geographical location, the applicable time, whether genders are to be combined. Providing misleading answers is not only unethical, it can have practical consequences. Too few services and facilities—which seriously disadvantages deaf people—or too sizable services and facilities—which wastes public moneys—can result from inaccurate demographic information.

Are there ways to overcome the difficulties inherent in attaining accurate, useful estimates of a deaf population? Yes, the methodological hurdle referred to by the U.S. Census Bureau has reference to the fact that in the 1830–1930 decennial censuses, each interviewer identified those they considered deaf. The Bureau acknowledged this problem but did not solve it.

Rather than leaving the definition of deafness up to each interviewer, I developed a Guttman-type scale to measure hearing. The Hearing Ability Scale (HAS) asks a series of questions that determine, by self-report, how each respondent hears.[11] Guttman scales are designed so that a reversal of responses—say, from yes to no—defines the quantity of what is being measured: For example, a series of questions to determine a respondent's weight might ask, Do you weigh more than 200 pounds? If the answer is no, the next question asks, Do you weigh more than 190 pounds? If no, then 180 pounds? When the person answers yes, the weight has been determined within 10 pounds.[12] In the same way, responses to HAS assess the respondent's ability to hear.

The National Health Survey has used HAS for 35 years. In the initial research, HAS correlated highly with audiometrics.[13] Researchers in the United Kingdom found it yielded results almost identical to those in the United States—an astonishingly close cross-validation of a verbal instrument administered in two different countries.[14]

TABLE 2.4   The Hearing Ability Scale (HAS)

Instructions read to respondent: Please answer each of the next questions the way you usually hear with both ears. If you use a hearing aid please answer the way you hear without the aid.

1. Can you usually hear and understand what a person says without seeing his face if he whispers to you from across a quiet room?
2. Can you usually hear and understand what a person says without seeing his face if he talks to you in a normal voice from across a quiet room?
3. Can you usually hear and understand what a person says without seeing his face if he shouts to you from across a quiet room?
4. Can you usually hear and understand what a person says if he speaks loudly into your better ear?
5. Can you usually tell the sound of speech from other sounds and noises?
6. Can you usually tell one kind of noise from another?
7. Can you hear loud noises?

Instructions to interviewer: Conclude questioning when respondent answers yes.

Source: Schein, J. D., & Delk, M. T. (1974). *The deaf population of the United States.* Silver Spring, MD: National Association of the Deaf.

Once the degree of hearing impairment is established demographers must consider other factors such as the ages at onset, the geographical locations of the persons sampled, and whatever additional characteristics are desired. They then report the distribution of the population sample's varying degrees of hearing impairment and ages at onset, as well as whatever characteristics have been ascertained. Such a report provides those receiving it with a broad picture of hearing impairment, recognizing, as it does, variations within the definition of deafness. Not all persons considered deaf have the same degree of hearing loss.

Will such procedures solve all demographic problems? No, there are the usual technical difficulties in determining the size and characteristics of any population—sampling being foremost among them. Our concern, however, has been those issues that are special for studies of hearing loss. For such studies, the obstacles are clear and some means for overcoming them have been discussed.

SOME CONCLUDING COMMENTS

The trouble with offhand guesstimates is that they inhibit efforts to obtain accurate, current information. Giving an answer implies that further studies are unnecessary. Government officials contend that more research on the deaf population is not needed, because they already have the information they need. That the data may be old, inaccurate, and incomplete does not deter them from defending that position; they have the answer!

Forty years ago, I attended a seminar at Gallaudet College intended to encourage psychologists to become involved with deaf persons. The first speaker concluded his remarks about the sociology of deafness and asked for questions. I asked, "How many deaf people are there?"

He promptly replied, "I don't know," and after a brief pause he added, "and neither does anyone else!"

His answer was ethical and, for its time, correct. The scattered studies that had been done were outdated and methodologically inadequate. His willingness to say, "I don't know" set an ethical standard for myself and I hope, for anyone seeking answers to demographic questions about deafness. Being ethical should not only command respect for good behavior; it should also be seen for its highly practical value. Honest answers prevent mistakes from occurring and encourage the search for accurate data—when they receive the attention they deserve.

REFERENCES

Goldstein, H., & Schein, J. D. (1964). Factors in the definition of deafness as they relate to incidence and prevalence. *Proceedings of the Conference on the Collection of Statistics of Severe Hearing Impairments and Deafness in the United States. March 19–20, 1964.* Public Health Service Publication No. 1227. Washington, DC: USGPO.

Levine, E. S. (1960). *The psychology of deafness.* New York: Columbia University Press.

Rainer, J. D., Altshuler, K. Z., Kallman, F. J., & Deming, W. E. (1963). *Family and mental problems in a deaf population.* New York: Department of Medical Genetics, New York State Psychiatric Institute. Columbia University.

Ries, P. W. (1992). Prevalence and characteristics of persons with hearing trouble, 1990–91. *Vital and Health Statistics, Series 10,* No. 103.

Schein, J. D. (1964). Factors in the definition of deafness as they relate to incidence and prevalence. In H. Goldstein & J. D. Schein (Eds.), *Proceedings of the Conference on the Collection of Statistics of Severe Hearing Impairments and Deafness in the United States, March 19–20, 1964.* Public Health Service Publication No. 1227. Washington, DC: USGPO.

Schein, J. D. (1968). *The Deaf community.* Washington, DC: Gallaudet College Press.

Schein, J. D. (1973). Hearing disorders. In L. T. Kurland, J. F. Kurtzke, & I. D. Goldberg (Eds.), *Epidemiology of neurologic and sense organ disorders* (pp. 276–304). Vital and Health Statistics Monographs, American Public Health Association. Cambridge, MA: Harvard University Press.

Schein, J. D. (1989). *At home among strangers.* Washington, DC: Gallaudet University Press.

Schein, J. D., Gentile, A., & Haase, K. (1970). Development and evaluation of an expanded hearing loss scale questionnaire. *Vital and Health Statistics, 2*(37), 23–29.

United States Bureau of the Census. (1931). *The blind and deaf-mutes in the United States: 1930.* Washington, DC: USGPO.

Ward, P. R., Tucker, A. M., Tudor, C. A., & Morgan, D. C. (1977). Self-assessment of hearing impairment: Test of the expanded Hearing Ability Scale Questionnaire on hearing impaired adults in England. *British Journal of Audiology, 11,* 33–39.

APPENDIX

Important or Main Points

- Essentially, ethics and the study of deaf demographics is individually defined by each demographer. Their definition most likely reflects the profession in which the demographer was trained, belongs to, or affiliates.

- The people with hearing losses who are being "counted" and the other "consumers" of deaf demographic data may have shifting reasons for wanting higher or lower figures in different circumstances. Money matters, provision and access to service, political gain, psychological "comfort" or assurance are a few factors that influence individuals or groups to desire certain demographic figures to be "found" and made known.
- The need for accurate demographic data cannot be underestimated, but defining deafness or even degree of hearing loss remains one of the key issues in accurately collecting demographic data.
- Demographics change with time. Changing birth rate, mortality rate, disease/illness, and migration patterns all contribute to changes in demographic findings over time.
- There is a difference between incidence and prevalence, and each has its place in any discussion of the demography of deafness. Incidence concerns the number of *new* cases of deafness at a given place in a given time. Prevalence concerns the *total number* of cases existing at a given place in a given time.
- Geography is an important factor in incidence and prevalence rates for deafness—the prevalence rate for each region in a country may differ from another and from that of the entire country. Thus, caution is needed when applying averages from large areas to their components.
- Demographic variables like age at onset of deafness, gender, economic status can all play roles in determining how to use the demographic data effectively.
- Guttman scales have been one approach that has proved useful over an extended period of time in collecting accurate demographic data.

Follow-up References or Suggestions

- For an extended discussion of deaf demographics in the United States, see Schein, J. D., & Delk, M. T. (1974). *The deaf population of the United States.* Silver Spring, MD: National Association of the Deaf.
- For an extended discussion of the demographics of Canadians with hearing impairments, see Schein, J. D. (1990). *Canadians with impaired hearing.* Ottawa, ON: Statistics Canada.
- For demographic information on the number of deaf and hard of hearing people in Israel, see Sela, I., & Weisel, A. (1992). *The Deaf community in Israel.* Tel Aviv, Israel: Association of the Deaf in Israel, National Insurance Institute, JDC Israel, Ministry of Labour and Social Affairs; and Statistical Abstract of Israel. (1993). Jerusalem: Bureau of Statistics.
- A search for information on demographics of deaf and hard of hearing people in Australia should start by contacting the Australian Bureau of Statistics at P.O. Box 10, Belconnen, ACT, 2615, and/or Australian Hearing at 126 Greville Street, Chatswood, NSW, 2067.

- Demographic data on deafness in the United Kingdom may be sought from the Medical Research Council's Institute of Hearing Research and the Office of Population Censuses and Surveys (OPCS). (See, for example, OPCS. (1988). *Survey of disability,* HMSO.)

Ethical Questions for Consideration

- Is there a basic level of support relative to a nation's demographic variables below which any discussion of deafness, education, and ethics is a waste of time since basic needs are not being met?
- Is the gap between known demographic realities and trends for provision of service relative to (a) political will, and (b) economic realities widening or narrowing?
- In the case of individuals who are deaf but have additional disabilities, is there a consistency in categorization for purpose of collecting demographic data? Or is it the case that in some instances categorization is on the basis of greatest deficit, and at other times no decision is made and they are all lumped into a "catch-all" category? Is there greater suffering under one of the conditions than the other?
- How often should demographic data on deafness be collected? Is every 10 years adequate? Would a more frequent data collection provide a diminishing return on investment?

NOTES

[1] This figure happens to match the U.S. National Health Survey's estimate of deaf and hard of hearing people, regardless of the age at onset, and including persons with tinnitus and temporary hearing losses. See Ries, P. W. (1992). Prevalence and characteristics of persons with hearing trouble, 1990–91. *Vital and Health Statistics, Series 10,* No. 103.

[2] Rainer, J. D., Altshuler, K. Z., Kallman, F. J., & Deming, W. E. (1963). *Family and mental problems in a deaf population.* New York: Department of Medical Genetics, New York State Psychiatric Institute, Columbia University.

[3] Levine, E. S. (1960). *The psychology of deafness.* New York: Columbia University Press.

[4] Goldstein, H., & Schein, J. D. (1964). Factors in the definition of deafness as they relate to incidence and prevalence. *Proceedings of the Conference on the Collection of Statistics of Severe Hearing Impairments and Deafness in the United States. March 19–20, 1964.* Public Health Service Publication No. 1227. Washington, DC: USGPO. See also, Schein, J. D. (1968). *The Deaf community.* Washington, DC: Gallaudet College Press.

[5] See page 2 of the U.S. Bureau of the Census. (1931). *The blind and deaf-mutes in the United States: 1930.* Washington, DC: United States Government Printing Office.

[6] Demographers distinguish between the number of new cases arising in a particular place and time (incidence) and the number of all cases existing at that place in a given time (prevalence). These are different numbers. Each has its place in any discussion of the demography of deafness. Incidence is important in uncovering trends, while prevalence reflects the current size of the deaf population. Even if incidence remains steady, the prevalence of deafness may increase because deaf people live longer than persons in general. Conversely, it would decrease if deaf people lived less long than per-

sons in general. Obviously, both estimates are subject to numerous factors. The reader can pursue others differentially affecting incidence and prevalence rates.

[7] Though the term offends many people, "deaf-mute" is commonly found in the older literature to refer to persons born deaf or, in some instances, deafened before the establishment of their speech. Throughout this text, we follow the accepted use of "prelingual deafness" to signify persons born deaf or deafened before 3 years of age.

[8] Amazonas is extremely poor, isolated in the Andes, while Callao is a relatively wealthy seaport where different gene pools frequently mix. For a detailed discussion about the potential causes of such wide variations, see Schein, J. D. (1973). Hearing disorders. In L. T. Kurland, J. F. Kurtzke, & I. D. Goldberg (Eds.), *Epidemiology of neurologic and sense organ disorders* (pp. 276–304). Vital and Health Statistics Monographs, American Public Health Association. Cambridge, MA: Harvard University Press.

[9] The common expression "age of onset" is mistaken, unless the user of that preposition means the onset's age. Age at onset is a shortened version of "the age of the individual at the time the condition occurred"—which is generally the intention of the phrase.

[10] Schein, J. D. (1989). *At home among strangers.* Washington, DC: Gallaudet University Press.

[11] Schein, J. D., Gentile, A., & Haase, K. (1970). Development and evaluation of an expanded hearing loss scale questionnaire. *Vital and Health Statistics, 2*(37), 23–39.

[12] Of course, one could ask questions in smaller or larger increments, depending on the accuracy desired.

[13] Schein, J. D., Gentile, A., & Haase, K. (1970). Development and evaluation of an expanded hearing loss scale questionnaire. *Vital and Health Statistics, 2*(37), 23–29.

[14] Ward, P. R., Tucker, A. M., Tudor, C. A., & Morgan, D. C. (1977). Self-assessment of hearing impairment: Test of the Expanded Hearing Ability Scale Questionnaire on hearing impaired adults in England. *British Journal of Audiology, 11,* 33–39.

3

DEAFNESS, SCIENCE, TECHNOLOGY, AND ETHICS

DES POWER[1]

AUTHOR INTRODUCTION

Des Power is Professor of Special Education and Director of the Centre for Deafness Studies and Research in the Faculty of Education at Griffith University in Brisbane, Australia. In this chapter his intent is to contrast medical and social-cultural models of deafness and the implications of each of those models for considering the ethical dimensions of existing and emerging technologies. These technologies include cochlear implants, hair cell regeneration, and genetic engineering, the use of all of which are supported by the proponents of a medical model of deafness. This medical model contrasts with sociocultural views of Deafness (and disabilities generally) as a "life condition" which, for those who inhabit it, provides a perfectly viable and comfortable life. The general community must decide if it can include Deafness (and other disabilities) within its definition of "the human condition" or whether it will need to eliminate Deafness as not conforming to a view of "normality." How a democratic society will decide on one of these courses is seen as a major ethical challenge for the near future.

CASES TO CONSIDER

What is the status of people with disabilities in our communities? How will we "see" them and live with them? Historically, people with disabilities have been unempowered in our societies by a common view that they are frustrated, unhappy individuals who are unable to play any part in "normal life" and who would wish to be "made whole" if they could be. We will examine this proposition at some length in this chapter, but the following two views of their own lives by "disabled" people present a very different perspective.

Simon Stevens is a severely cerebrally palsied Englishman. Here is his view of himself in an e-mail that was widely distributed. (Used here with permission from the author—secured 2000/11/21—original letter, message 89, dated 2000/08/31 may be found at http://www.clarity-network.com/):

> Dear all,
>
> My observations of the UK disability movement over the last few months and indeed years has shown a realization which I wish to share with everyone. My concerns became focused when I witnessed the debate on the film 'The Idiots'[2]. It seemed many disabled people argued that it was the moral duty of all disabled people to hate this film because it portrayed us in the wrong light, we never make a mess in public or wave our arms about.
>
> But the problem is I do make a mess in public and wave my arms about, that is a part of my impairment and therefore a part of me, and quite frankly I am proud of it! I am NOT normal and never want to be.
>
> So I realized that many disabled people, often those who have not faced oppression to any large degree, want to be normal and demand that all other disabled people should be normal, not in a biological way but in a social way. The social model, in its most pure form, is normalization, it is the medical model for social normality. I am not arguing against the social model since I do not believe it is as pure as it was and is now a symbolic model for power, access, etc. Plus it is developing and concepts of impairment, identity and pride have a place.
>
> So is the disabled movement about normalization? Well, some parts are and I would challenge many disability academics to argue they are not into normalization? My realization is the disabled movement is not about structures and powers but more about a force (like Star Wars) and a change coming from individuals, groups, organizations etc. E-mail is playing a large part in building a stronger disability movement; this e-mail may reach a large population of people active in disability.
>
> So as you guess I hate normalization in all its forms. I believe we are seeing the start of a new element of disability/impairment politics: pride and self-expression. I am not sure if this means the self-oppressive arts and poetry I sometimes see but something more positive. I am not proud of my oppression but I am proud of who I am and I wish to express to the world who that is, a bib-wearing, helmet-wearing dribbling spastic that talks funny, waves everything about and makes a mess wherever he goes!
>
> I have met many people who share my pride in themselves and desire not to be normal, whatever that damn word means. I do feel a new stronger movement is being built right now, by me, by my friends and colleagues, by people I am yet to meet and by people I may never meet! I doubt that there will ever be a formal structure to the movement but rather through e-mail and personal contact, this movement will grow by not just having people but knowing people, sharing oppressive expressives and being open about who we are.
>
> Therefore the normalization bible should be burnt as we begin to discover ourselves and become true allies in achieving the right thing, which may include taking the piss out of ourselves at times.
>
> This is my waffle and just an opinion so no burst veins please!

My second example is from an anonymous Deaf man reported by De Matteo, Lou, and Burke (1990). In a clinical setting a Deaf man was presented with the traditional game of a "Good Fairy" appearing and granting him three wishes—whatever he desired. His first wish was for more interpreting support to be easily available, the second for more understanding of Deafness as a cultural and linguistic phenomenon, and the third was for more captioned television. When asked why he would not ask to become hearing, he said, "But then I wouldn't be *me!*"

People with disabilities are often comfortable with the lives they have made—they would not wish to be otherwise, difficult though their lives in a nonaccepting or nonunderstanding community may sometimes be.

INTRODUCTION

In *The Birth of the Modern* Paul Johnson (1991, p. 1000) quotes Charles Lamb writing to a friend in 1830 deploring the rise of Science, "Can we ring the bells backwards? ... There is a march of Science. But who shall beat the drums for its retreat?" Johnson's epigrammatic answer to Lamb's question was, "Answer came there none, nor ever could." There appears to be no stopping the march of Science and its handmaiden, Technology. What is not so clear is whether society's understanding of the ethical challenges created by advances in science and technology and the will to shape social and political answers to those challenges has kept pace. Recent developments in "deafness technology" such as cochlear implants, cochlear hair cell regeneration (Marzella & Clark, 1999), and particularly in genetic knowledge arising from the Human Genome Project and the genetic engineering that will follow (Davila, 2000), with their promise of intervening in vitro or in utero to manipulate the characteristics of the developing individual present a never-before-faced challenge to our appreciation of "the human condition"—a challenge to our very understanding of what it means to be human and of the status of human life.

Davila (2000) reflected on these technologies, especially genetic screening with its promise of intervening to manipulate developing individual's characteristics to achieve the perfect baby. He, like others, has raised his hands and voice to the challenge of appreciating the varied human condition. He wondered about what it means to be human and the importance of life if deafness is to be considered something that needs to be manipulated out of existence.

The challenge faces not only those concerned with deafness. It is already possible to detect the presence of Down syndrome and many other conditions caused by genetic "defects" early enough in pregnancy to allow abortion to be considered; doubtless similar early tests for hearing loss in utero will soon be available too. Simple blood tests can detect more and more genetic conditions (including hereditary hearing impairment) in utero (some 400 in 1999, according to Parens & Asch) and the technology to "engineer" changes in genetic structure to prevent these conditions being manifested is already available and growing in range and sophistication almost daily.

THE QUESTION OF "NORMALITY" AND "DISABILITY"

The possibilities of intervening described earlier present us with difficult decisions not only about life and death (in deciding whether a fetus detected early enough should be aborted), but about what it means for human life to be "normal" and about the nature of "disability" itself. What will be considered normal—and who will decide? Who is disabled and who will decide? Is "normality" necessary or even desirable (should society be able to bear [and even celebrate] a wide range of normality)? Who may be included in the "normal" and "disabled" categories? Is deafness a "disability"?[3] None of these are new questions, but they are no longer hypothetical.

Many (particularly prelingually) Deaf people do not see themselves as "disabled" and argue that deafness is just another aspect of normality—they are "normal," they just happen not to be able to hear.[4] While they may have a "biophysical maladaption" (in Hughes' [2000] phrase) any disability they have is "socially constructed" and a result of the physical and attitudinal barriers that a noncomprehending society imposes upon them (Power, 1992; 1997; also see Gregory & Hartley, 1991 and Higgins & Nash, 1987. For disability generally, see Parens & Asch, 1999).[5] For the purposes of the present discussion, it is helpful to consider the literature concerning disability more generally and the ethical issues raised therein, especially in the context of what Vehmas (1999) has called the "bioutilitarian ethics" of Singer (1981; 1993), Kuhse and Singer (1985), Kuhse (1987, 1995), and Rachels (1986). Through Hughes (2000) we can link bioutilitarian ethics to the "medical" view of disability which Hughes sees as being responsible for the "aestheticisation" of attitudes to disability. The medical view of disability (and of life generally) is "offended" by biophysical maladaptation and the genetic and other technologies are being driven to delete from humankind any individuals who do not confirm to the "norm" of "soundness" (and perhaps even beauty too). Such beliefs may constitute a real danger for people with disabilities—certainly as far as any amelioration of societal attitudes toward disability is concerned (see Parens & Asch, 1999, for a particularly useful review), and even, in the case of fetuses determined to be "maladapted" by some criterion, to life itself. On utilitarian (what Vehmas, 1999, has also called "intelligist") grounds it is already permissible (and even encouraged) to abort fetuses demonstrated to be "suffering" from Down syndrome, muscular dystrophy, neural tube defects, and other abnormalities detected early in pregnancy. Within utilitarian and aestheticization ethics where might this pressure for normalization cease? Will deafness be included in reasons for abortion or genetic engineering when it can be detected early enough? As Ramsay (1994) says,

> The boundaries of what is genetically desirable and what is undesirable will change in accordance with the values[6] of those who select the criteria for what counts as a genetic defect or handicap. The classification of defects may be based on subjective and ideological beliefs about the costs and benefits to society, the value or availability of certain qualities or characteristics. What is not perfect has limitless boundaries if it ever became possible for designer genes to reflect the latest fashion and determine what kind of future people there could be. (p. 254)

We have been down that slippery slope before, and we know where it leads—to eugenics and the politicization of decisions about who will live or die or be engineered into the kind of beings considered desirable for society. ("Lessons from a dark and dangerous past" as Müller-Hill, 1994, called them).

As a number of authors have observed: If the technology is there, it will inevitably be used.

PATHS AND LIVES-LIVED

Whatever one's social or religious beliefs about abortion, a pause for thought must be taken if it was suggested that a fetus be aborted because of genetic deafness—given that we know that a perfectly viable life can be established as a deaf or Deaf individual (Hyde & Power, 2000. Also see Higgins & Nash, 1987; Gregory & Hartley, 1991; National Association of the Deaf, 2000; Power, 1997). It is clear that a "Deaf life" is not "a life not worth living" in bioutilitarian terms and disposal of such lives cannot be justified on those grounds.

Vehmas (1999) has made the point that there are serious flaws in the bioutilitarian approach, even in the context of severe intellectual disability. The bioutilitarians argue that such a life is "not worth living," but as Vehmas has said,

> A perfect existence is beyond the reach of human beings. If a full human life is … defined as pursuing successfully some possibilities which are good or the best which restricted human reality offers, it would not matter if an individual had restricted possibilities, and, it could be argued that many people do live a full human life. … The morality … [of bioutilitarianism] is based upon some vague concept of normality and, as a result, what we have is a hopelessly relativistic basis for moral judgements [such as whether a "biologically maladapted" infant shall live or die] (p. 43). … Individuals determine their own interests and their own criteria for a satisfactory life. (p. 45)

Who will decide what the criteria are? Will we screen out future possible Stephen Hawkings or Helen Kellers or Christy Browns, the central figure in the book "My Left Foot"? What of the Oscar-winning Deaf actress Marlee Matlin or the deaf Miss America Heather Whitestone or the "supercrips" of the Paralympics, or our dribbling, arm-waving man describing himself earlier—and many, many others like them? Where will we draw the line? How much would the variety of human life lose if such individuals were lost to us? Everyone has a life to live on their own terms and society has a responsibility to ameliorate those lives that are not entirely satisfactory to those who live them.

How much more true is this of a deaf/Deaf life! As Hughes (2000, p. 561; quoting Glassner, 1992) has put it, we must not be subject to the "tyranny of perfection" in these matters. In the end, as Duster (1990; quoted by Parsons & Bradley, 1994) has remarked, "Genetic research and screening for genetic disorders have the potential for doing great amounts of good and great amounts of harm. The way in which human societies … move into this arena will be shaped as much by social forces as by concerns for the general public health" (p. 95). Again, Sinclair and Griffiths (1994), "Social attitudes of discrimination and exclusion [can be, and] must not be created or reinforced by social policy, or be reflected in present or future legislation. Ethical questions must be addressed alongside scientific ones. The power to do something does not justify it or make it the right thing to do" (p. 206).

We must be aware of these "social forces" and be sure that they are thoroughly debated and brought to public awareness before nonreversible decisions are made about what lives are worth preserving and what "biological maladaptations" (such as deafness) fall within an acceptable range of "normal human differences."

Hughes lays much of the problems facing people with disabilities (including, in this context, deaf/Deaf people) at the feet of the medical model of disability, and states that,

> While the medical model demands that disabled people adapt to society, the social model [the "socially constructed life" model described earlier] demands changes in social structure that will reflect the needs of disabled [read "Deaf"] people. The social model emphasises the collective, structural, and social—as opposed to the individual, personal and medical—origins of disability (p. 556) … Medical distinctions are powerful cultural distinctions which promote and reinforce social hierarchies and sort people into the bare "essentials" of humanity. (p. 558)

In other words, medical models are just as much socially constructed as are social models, and, as such can, and should, be amenable to "social reconstruction" in the light of a better understanding of the social nature of disability.[7] What is required is not the force-fitting of people with disabilities into categories of mal-adaptation. Rather, what is required is a better understanding on the part of the medical and other professions, the media, and the public of the "true nature" of disabled lives and the role social institutions can play in making those lives viable, enjoyable, and fruitful for whatever purposes people with disabilities wish to make of them. As Ferguson (quoted by Parens & Asch, 1999) has said, "The challenge is to create the society that will allow as many different paths as possible to the qualities of life that make us all part of the human community" (p. 14).

IMPLANTS AND GENETICS AND REGENERATION

I have couched the preceding discussion mainly in terms of likely developments in genetic screening and genetic engineering of in vitro or in utero development, but even if deafness avoids genetic engineering or abortion (because of the difficulty of diagnosis of deafness in utero) ethical issues are beginning to arise after birth in the context of the use of the cochlear implant technology, and probably will with the future availability of restoration of hearing via cochlear hair-cell regeneration. I refer not so much to general ethics of the use of pharmaceutical restoration of hair cells or cochlear implant technology and accompanying surgery to "cure" a non-life-threatening condition such as deafness, which Deaf associations have been so opposed to (Australian Association of the Deaf, n.d.; Hyde & Power, 2000; Victorian Council of Deaf People, 1991),[8] or to whether parents have the right to decide for their young deaf child whether to have an implant fitted (clearly they do; Hyde & Power, 2000; National Association of the Deaf, 2000), but to issues surrounding the acceptance (or not) by affected parties of the "ameliorating" effects of technology. The movie *Gattaca* has already portrayed a time when refusal to accept a genetically engineered fate may become illegal, with social and legal sanctions for refusal. In the context of a paper on cochlear implants, and with the Deaf community's position clearly in mind, Tucker (1998) reviewed a number of U.S. court decisions where it was held that individuals refusing ameliorating surgery after (say) motor accidents have been refused insurance cover for other costs arising out of claimed continuing disability. Tucker speculates that public funding support might not be forthcoming in the future for special education services for children whose parents refuse the possibly beneficial effects of an implant.

> It seems likely that in the future more courts will hold that the law does not require that an individual with a physical impairment be provided with accommodations which would be necessary if the individual would obtain reasonable medical treatment that would obviate the need for such accommodations. ... Members of the public, including politicians, are likely to ask: why should the public and private sectors be required to spend money to provide accommodations for a person whose disability is correctable, when correcting the disability would in itself help level the playing field for that person? (Tucker, p. 12)

In the context of prenatal testing for disabling conditions Parens and Asch (1999) have strongly put forward the alternative view. We can place their statement in the context of Tucker's quoted earlier about refusing "possibly ameliorating treatments" such as cochlear implants.

> Policies that would in any way penalize those who continue pregnancies in spite of knowing that their child will live with a disabling trait must be avoided. Those prospective parents who either forgo prenatal testing or decide that they want to continue a pregnancy despite the detection of a disabling trait should not have to contend with losing medical services or benefits for their child, nor feel obliged to justify their decisions. Further, the availability of prenatal testing in no way reduces our societal obligations to those people who are born with or acquire disabilities. (pp. 4–5)[9]

Hyde and Power (2000), in commenting on Tucker's position, have said that it will clearly become crucial how "reasonable medical treatment" and whether a disability is "correctable" or not are to be defined and who is going to do the defining. As they have pointed out, if the cochlear implant is considered "reasonable medical treatment" (and the present definer of this, the medical profession, believes that it is), and if the implant can be considered to provide "correction" (and the evidence is presently that some child implant recipients do so benefit; though some do not), how is this to be determined, and by whom? Consider the reality of how parents, mostly "new" to deafness, are to have sufficient information to make a "fully informed choice" about whether or not their child should have an implant. Hyde and Power and the National Association of the Deaf (2000) have argued that, for parental choice to be fully informed, the risk/benefit/choice model presented to parents must be broadened to include the social, linguistic, and cultural aspects of the possibilities of a "viable Deaf life": a life that includes the rich personal, social, cultural, and linguistic context that membership of the Deaf community could provide. Without a doubt, parents of deaf children should have such information available if they are to be fully informed about the futures possible for their child (I would now add, with or without an implant; cf. Bahan's movement toward the possibility of viewing the implant as just another kind of hearing aid. See Endnote 5).

Hyde and Power (2000) have demonstrated that in a typical cochlear implant program in Australia, these requirements of fully informed consent are not usually met. Informed consent appears to be focused on "risk criteria" that are narrowly medical and, indeed, concentrate on protecting medical providers against negligence claims due to not entirely satisfactory outcomes of the medical procedure.[10] Hyde and Power comment that, "The informed consent procedures were determined by the medical provider, administered by the medical provider and final authorization for fitting managed by the medial provider, ... and included only the medical parameters of benefit and risk, not the personal, social or educational ones [or, on the other hand, the possible benefits of a 'deaf life']" (p. 123).

As Parsons and Bradley (1994) have said, "What makes consent 'informed'? It is important that the individual knows the facts and that there is an understanding of the relevant issues" (p. 103).

> The yearning for the certainty of absolutes [such as the "perfect nonbiologically-maladapted individual"] has resulted historically not in justice or equality or liberty but in the denial of moral personhood to all those categories of living beings who cannot be identified in terms of the ideal standard. (Shildrick, 1997, p. 212)

CONCLUSIONS

There is a strong tendency to see the condition instead of the person and to deny "moral personhood" to people who are deaf by insisting that deafness is a condition to be "cured." Society must face up to some complex ethical and sociopolitical decisions about the matters canvassed previously before it is too late and we are swamped by the ongoing march of science and technology. We may not be able to stay their march, but we must be aware of the implications of allowing them to go forward.

REFERENCES

Australian Association of the Deaf. (n.d.). *Policy on the cochlear implant.* Petersham: Australian Association of the Deaf.

Davila, R. (2000). *Education of the Deaf in the new millennium: Assessing the past and projecting into the future.* Keynote Address, International Congress on Education of the Deaf. Sydney: The Australian Association of Teachers of the Deaf.

Davis, L. J. (1995). *Enforcing normalcy: Disability, deafness, and the body.* New York: Verso.

De Matteo, A. J., Lou, M. W., & Burke, F. (1990). *The impact of deafness on development.* Paper presented at Grand Rounds, Department of Psychiatry, University of California San Francisco.

Glassner, B. (1992). *Bodies: The tyranny of perfection.* Los Angeles: Lowell House.

Gregory, S., & Hartley, G. (Eds.). (1991). *Constructing deafness.* London: Pinter.

Gross, N. E. (1985). *Everyone here spoke sign language: Hereditary deafness on Martha's Vineyard.* Cambridge, MA: Harvard University Press.

Higgins, P., & Nash, J. (Eds.). (1987). *Understanding deafness socially.* Springfield, IL: C. C. Thomas.

Hughes, B. (2000). Medicine and the aesthetic invalidation of disabled people. *Disability & Society, 15,* 555–568.

Hyde, M., & Power, D. (2000). Informed parental consent for cochlear implantation of young deaf children: Social and other considerations in the use of the "Bionic Ear." *Australian Journal of Social Issues, 35,* 117–128.

Johnson, P. (1991). *The birth of the modern.* New York: HarperCollins.

Johnson, R. C. (2000). Gallaudet forum addresses cochlear implant issues. *Research at Gallaudet, Spring 2000.* Washington, DC: Gallaudet University, Gallaudet Research Institute.

Kuhse, H. (1987). *The sanctity-of-life doctrine in medicine: A critique.* Oxford: Clarendon Press.

Kuhse, H. (1995). Quality of life as a decision-making criterion. In A. Goldsworth, W. Silverman, D. K. Stevenson, E. W. D. Young, & R. Rivers (Eds.), *Ethics and perinatology.* New York: Oxford University Press.

Kuhse, H., & Singer, P. (1985). *Should the baby live? The problem of handicapped infants.* Oxford: Oxford University Press.

Marzella, P. L., & Clark, G. M. (1999). Growth factors, auditory neurones and cochlear implants: A review. *Acta Oto-Laryngologica, 119,* 407–412.

Müller-Hill, B. (1994). Lessons from a dark and distant past. In A. Clarke (Ed.), *Genetic counselling: Practice and principles* (pp. 133–141). London: Routledge.

National Association of the Deaf. (2000). *NAD position statement on cochlear implants* [On-line]. Available: http://www.nad.org/infocenter/newsroom/papers/CochlearImplants.html.

Parens, E., & Asch, A. (1999). The disability rights critique of prenatal genetic testing: Reflections and recommendations. *Hastings Center Report, September–October, Special Supplement.*

Parsons, E., & Bradley, D. (1994). Ethical issues in newborn screening for Duchenne muscular dystrophy: The question of informed consent. In A. Clarke (Ed.), *Genetic counselling: Practice and principles* (pp. 95–112). London: Routledge.

Power, D. (1992). Deaf people: A linguistic and cultural minority or a disability group? *Australian Disability Review,* 4–92, 43–48.

Power, D. (1997). *Constructing lives: The Deaf experience.* Brisbane: Griffith University, Faculty of Education.

Pueschel, S. M. (1991). Ethical considerations relating to prenatal diagnosis of fetuses with Down syndrome. *Mental Retardation, 29*(4), 185–190.

Rachels, J. (1986). *The end of life: Euthanasia and morality.* Oxford: Oxford University Press.

Ramsay, M. (1994). Genetic reductionism and medical genetᵢc practice. In A. Clarke (Ed.), *Genetic counselling: Practice and principles* (pp. 241–260). London: Routledge.

Shildrick, M. (1997). *Leaky bodies and boundaries: Feminism, postmodernism and (bio)ethics.* London: Routledge.

Sinclair, L., & Griffiths, M. (1994). Medical genetics and mental handicap. In A. Clarke (Ed.), *Genetic counselling: Practice and principles.* London: Routledge.

Singer, P. (1981). *The expanding circle: Ethics and sociobiology.* Oxford: Clarendon Press.

Singer, P. (1993). *Practical ethics* (2nd ed.). Cambridge: Cambridge University Press.

Stevens, S. (2000). *Normalisation vs pride and self-expression* [On-line]. Available: http://www.clarity-network.com/.

Tucker, B. (1998). Deaf culture, cochlear implants, and elective disability. *Hastings Center Report, 28*(4), 6–14.

Vehmas, S. (1999). Discriminative assumptions of utilitarian bioethics regarding individuals with intellectual disabilities. *Disability & Society, 14,* 37–52.

Victorian Council of Deaf People. (1991). *Cochlear implant policy.* Melbourne: Victorian Council of Deaf People.

APPENDIX

Important or Main Points

- Science and technology continue to progress and develop—some areas related to deafness include cochlear implants, hair-cell regeneration, the study of genetics, and even genetic intervening. Whether social policy and political answers have kept pace is a critical area.
- Deafness may be viewed biophysically or socially constructed. In the first, a loss of hearing is described as a disability. In the second the deafness is seen as just another aspect or variation of normality.
- A "deaf/Deaf life" is a perfectly viable life. An individual with a hearing loss has the potential like any other person to fully participate in life-roles—to become educated, employed, establish relationships, parent, contribute to society, etc. If these larger life roles are featured, then the disposal or termination of a life that may have a hearing loss cannot be justified on bioutilitarian terms.
- Positive change could be initiated for those with a biophysical background by fostering a greater exposure and a better understanding into the true nature of disabled lives, the role institutions can play in providing "good lives," and what the disabled themselves think.
- Informed consent is often inadequate—from the perspective of parents being informed and understanding all the options. In the case of cochlear implants, too often the consent is limited to the relatively short-term medical implications of the surgery and post-implant therapy.

Follow-up References or Suggestions

- Although dated for some information, parents may still be interested in the "professional point of view" and the "life stories" of parents and children with hearing losses as they made decisions about communication approaches, as contained in Schwartz, S. (Ed.). (1987). *Choices in deafness: A parents guide: Cued speech: Oral approach: Total communication.* Washington, DC: Woodbine House.
- Raskind, M. H., & Higgins, E. L. (1995). Reflections on ethics, technology and learning disabilities: Avoiding the consequences of ill-considered actions. *Journal of Learning Disabilities, 28*(7), 425–438.
- Information on Genetics and Deafness

  1. American Society of Human Genetics/American Board of Medical Genetics, 9650 Rockville Pike, Bethesda, MD, 20814. Phone (301) 571–1925.
  2. Genetic Services Center, Gallaudet University, 800 Florida Ave. NE, Washington, DC, 20002. Phone (202) 651-5258 (voice/TDD), or (800) 451–8834, ext. 5258 (voice/TDD).
  3. March of Dimes Birth Defects Foundation, Professional Education, 1275 Mamaroneck Ave., White Plains, NY, 10605.

4. National Society of Genetic Counselors, 233 Canterbury Dr., Wallingford, PA, 19086. Phone (215) 872–7608.

- Bioethics and disability was the focus of two issues of *Interaction,* the journal of the National Council on Intellectual Disability in Australia.

  1. NCID. (2000). Bioethics and disability. *Interaction, 13*(3), 3–32, C. Newell (Guest Editor). This issue contains an article concerning ethics, deafness, and implants: Newell, C. "Access to opportunity or oppression? An Australian policy analysis of the ethics of the cochlear implant."
  2. NCID. (2000). Bioethics and disability II. *Interaction, 13*(4), 3–33, C. Newell (Guest Editor).

Ethical Questions for Consideration

- Davila (2000) highlighted that one of the possible long-term outcomes from the Human Genome project would include the production of the "perfect" baby on a regular basis—that is, that gene therapy could lead to a substantial reduction in deafness. Still, Davila wondered whether this would be possible until the ethical issues (examined previously) are resolved.
- It is possible to only speculate at this time on the "progress" of hair-cell regeneration. First to possibly minimize the profound effects of diseases like meningitis. Second to possibly repair longer-standing hearing loss due to cell damage from other things like disease/noise/trauma. And finally, to consider "initiating" hearing from those who have an absence of hair cells in the cochlea from birth. Are the ethics of "acceptance" in one possibility different from the others?
- Surgical interventions on the unborn to correct a recognized life-threatening condition have occurred. Certainly, in these instances the case is clearer. The issue for "correcting" a nonlife-threatening defect is unlikely to be as clearcut—especially when the risks to the mother and unborn child are considered. Where should the "line in the sand" be drawn?
- Are there more tolerant societies/cultures that accept or even embrace "difference" or disabilities? If there are—where are they? Can we learn from them? Do the developed nations show the most tolerance or the least? Deaf culture is certainly more tolerant of deafness, but does this carry over to mental retardation or other physical or sensory deformities?
- Quality of life research is becoming very popular—even in the area of cochlear implantation. See for example, the (2000) article "Cost-utility analysis of the cochlear implant in children" in the *Journal of the American Medical Association, 284*(7). Do the "measurement tools" used in this type of research represent a broad enough church for what constitutes "quality of life" to make pronouncements? Is the financial cost-benefit weighting over emphasized?
- In ancient times physically deformed infants were killed or abandoned at birth, but some deaf and blind children may have missed that fate because of

the invisibility of their defect. Later in the child's life the parents may have become too attached to the infant to "throw it to the wolves" when the defect was finally discovered. Is the ancient dilemma and the modern dilemma the same—albeit conducted at an early stage of the child's life because of advances in testing for identification?

NOTES

[1] I am grateful to Rod Beattie and Linus Power for helpful comments on the development of this chapter.

[2] This is a 1998 film made in Denmark by Lars von Trier who was the writer, director, and cinematographer. The following (1999) quotation is from Sabadino Parker, PopMatters Film Critic [Online]. Available: http://popmatters.com/film/reviews/i/idiots.html. The film is an

> ...exploration of normality as a social system, the constraints it places on individuals to behave in prescribed ways even under abnormal circumstances. The film chronicles the escapades of a small group of young middle-class men and women who have formed an organization to upset what they perceive to be bourgeois principles and participants, that is, well-to-do and unscrupulous people. The group attempts to accomplish its goals by acting as if they are mentally challenged, so as to annoy the gentlefolk with their "spassing" (spastic behavior), and interacting with each other within the confines of their private commune.

[3] As Davis (1995) has pointed out in discussing the historical construction of deafness, disability and normalcy, the very concepts of "normality" and "disability" in their modern sense are quite recent sociopolitical constructions of the eighteenth and nineteenth centuries.

[4] What is also coming to be called "the wellness model" of deafness (National Association of the Deaf, 2000).

[5] This issue is complex. Parens and Asch (1999) have made a useful point that "disability" is in fact not "neutral" or "normal" —

> the societal provision of special resources and services to people with disabilities depends on noticing the descriptive and evaluative senses in which disabling traits are not neutral, and how the needs of the people who live with them are, descriptively speaking, not normal. Yet the recognition of the obligation to provide those special resources is rooted in a commitment to the fundamental idea that the people living with those traits are, morally speaking, "normal"; the people bearing the traits are evaluatively normal in the sense of deserving the normal respect due equally to all persons. (p. 15)

Parens and Asch then continue:

> Unequal or special funding expresses a commitment to moral equality. Recognizing the non-neutrality of the trait and the "ab-normality" of the person's needs is necessary for expressing the commitment to moral equity and equal opportunity. There is nothing paradoxical about appreciating the descriptive sense in which people with disabling traits are abnormal while also appreciating the evaluative or moral sense in which they are normal. (p. 15)

[6] And, one should add, the knowledge and social status of those who make the decisions. There is ample evidence, for example, that high socioeconomic status better-educated women are more likely to access genetic screening and there are differing rates of deciding whether or not to have an abortion of a (say) Down syndrome fetus according to social class and education level. (For a "survey" discussion see Pueschel, 1991 and listed references.) It is also evident that for a considerable time, genetic screening will be a "luxury" of developed nations. Parents in the developing nations are unlikely to be able to avail themselves of it. Major inequalities in these matters appear at all turns.

[7] And, indeed have been, as Gross (1985) has shown how significant numbers of Deaf people were a normal part of a mixed hearing/Deaf community on Martha's Vineyard in the nineteenth century.

[8] Though some easing of these strong positions may be beginning, if the reported views of Bahan (in Johnson, 2000), a well-known Deaf writer and activist and father of two deaf children, are indicative,

> Conflicting perceptions about implants … have put the deaf community and the medical community on an apparent collision course for many years, but … this appearance may be the result of misconceptions about implants. When implants are seen as capable of changing deaf people into hearing people, members of the deaf community naturally see them as threats to their cultural identities. When viewed as devices that can help make the hearing world more accessible to deaf people … implants appear more like hearing aids, devices which deaf Americans, by and large, have come to accept. (p. 7)

Bahan suggests that if,

> [. . .] deaf children with implants are allowed to use sign language and maintain contact with other deaf people, then implants may be seen simply as helping them enlarge their scope of awareness without destroying their identities as deaf people. (p. 7)

The most recent statement by the (American) National Association of the Deaf (2000) also indicates some softening of the former hard line against child implantation taken by the Association.

[9] But there are straws in the wind. What of the following report from *The Australian* (2000, November 20):

> PARIS: France's highest court ruled in a landmark case on Saturday that a youth born with severe handicaps could demand compensation for being born rather than being aborted. Josette and Christian Perruche, parents of the deaf, retarded and nearly blind 17-year-old Nicholas, won their appeal for compensation on the grounds that doctors should have prevented his birth.

[10] Typical "Possible risks" Statement from an Australian Cochlear Implant Program (Hyde & Power, 2000):

1. Inability to place some or all of the electrodes inside the cochlea.
2. Infection at the site of the surgery, perhaps requiring the removal of the device.
3. Leakage of fluid from the cochlea, perhaps requiring a further operation.
4. Electronic failure of the cochlear implant.
5. Injury to the facial nerve, causing either temporary or permanent facial "weakness."
6. Disturbance of taste.
7. Giddiness.
8. Increased tinnitus.
9. Unsuccessful electrical stimulation, due to insufficient hearing nerve fibers.
10. Some electrodes may stimulate non-hearing nerves, causing pain or discomfort.
11. Should there be a need for the patient [sic] to undergo Magnetic Resonance Imaging the magnet in the cochlear implant would need to be surgically removed.

And, the final additions to the possible risks list were,

- In addition to the preceding, some risks are involved in general anesthesia: chest, heart, and brain complications may occur.
- The procedure may also involve risks that are currently not known.
- No compensation will be provided as no more than minimal risk is involved.

4

MOTHER TONGUE/FIRST LANGUAGE

DEENA M. MARTIN, MICHAEL RODDA, AND
SUSANNE MARTIN

AUTHOR INTRODUCTION

This chapter has been brought together through the efforts of three individuals from the Western Canadian Center for Studies in Deafness. Dr. Rodda, who is presently the director of the Center, is also a professor at the University of Alberta and the holder of the David Piekoff Chair of Deafness Studies. He has spent much of his academic career researching and teaching on the topic of language development, mental health, and deafness. Susanne Martin has her undergraduate degree in Education from the University of Alberta and a master's degree in counseling from Gonzaga University. She has also worked in the field of deafness as a certified American Sign Language Interpreter for 25 years. Her extensive experience working with families and deafness has resulted in valuable examples found throughout the chapter. And finally, Deena Martin is presently working on her masters in Educational Psychology, specializing in Deafness. She has nine years of experience in working in rehabilitation settings with Deaf and hard of hearing clients and other disabled people.

The intent of this introduction was to introduce ourselves along with any biases that we may bring to the chapter. Perhaps the most fundamental bias that needs to be identified is our commitment to individual choice and the right to receive the information necessary to make informed decisions about our needs, our lives, and our strategies for resolving problems. We are deeply committed to the belief that all individuals and families, regardless of ability/disability and socioeconomic status, have these rights. Deafness and language development, as discussed in the chapter, is an area that is surrounded by opposing perspectives, feuding special interest groups, and overwhelming confusion. The best decision is not one made by the professionals, but one made by the family. Each family/client, however, requires information provided in a manner that is understandable and unbiased. In this chapter, it was our intent to explore the ethical considerations that surround the decision of choosing a first language for a deaf child. Whether you are a professional or a parent, we hope that this chapter provides you with a unique perspective into deafness and language development.

A CASE TO CONSIDER

Casey is a 10-year-old, Caucasian male, residing with his mother in urban Canada. He attends a local segregated school for the deaf and participates in community events during the evenings and weekends. At school, Casey receives instruction in American Sign Language (ASL) for the majority of his classes. He was, however, recently introduced to Signed English to assist him with reading comprehension. In the home, Casey's mother and father use ASL. After Casey's diagnosis, his parents attended ASL classes (taught by local Deaf instructors) to ensure successful communication with Casey. At this time, however, they are not fluent.

Casey is a bright, energetic student who has become frustrated and is slowly withdrawing from others. His concerned mother fears that his lack of achievement in reading and writing is affecting his self-confidence and willingness to interact with others. Consequently, his mother has sought the support of the professionals to assist her in helping her son. After extensive testing, it is clear that Casey in an exceptionally clever boy with an above average intelligence. Yet, this seems to contrast sharply with his academic achievement in reading and writing. Despite receiving one-to-one assistance, he has not progressed past a reading level of grade two. What is happening?

To understand Casey and his connection to his community, it is essential that we examine his perceptual skills and ability to make sense of the world. Beginning with his home environment, Casey has been using "home" signs and ASL to communicate his needs and desires with his family. This language code has been successfully carried over to his school environment, where he has the opportunity to interact with Deaf adult role models and increase his signing skills. At school, Casey is also learning to read and write using Signed English (to assist in learning word order). In the community, Casey uses a type of home sign that is made up by he and his friends—a child's attempt to decrease the communication barrier. Because Casey is exceptionally bright, it can be assumed that he has his own inner understanding of the world. With all of these fragmented language codes one is left asking how he makes sense of his world if he does not have one language code in which he is fluent and able to communicate with others.

INTRODUCTION TO LANGUAGE

What is language? How does language influence one's belonging and acceptance into a community? How does a family choose a first language for a child with a severe hearing loss? How can a family prevent their child from experiencing Casey's situation? It is the intent of this chapter to assist the family and professionals in exploring the ethical complexity surrounding the decision of first language. This chapter will not provide an answer about which language model is ideal; instead its goal is to provide meaningful discourse that will create awareness and promote discussion.

Historical Perspective on Language

Exploring the evolution of deafness education is important to understanding the profound effect of promoting ethical decision-making practices on behalf of both the parents and the professionals.

Aristotle, Hippocrates, Plato, Darwin—many of the world's greatest philosophers pondered the concept and origin of language. Language and special education interventions are age-old controversies that have prevailed (unresolved) from century to century. In an insightful article titled "A Tale Often Told: The Early Progression of Special Education," Winzer (1998) describes how Spain was developing special education programs to teach those with severe multiple disabilities in the late sixteenth century. In 1578, Pedro Ponce de Leon initiated one of the first formal attempts at educating the deaf. Interestingly, Winzer explains that this attempt was more about the wealthy and the strict inheritance statutes rather than the philosophical nature of language development. In the seventeenth century, documentation reveals that British "researchers" began teaching their "subjects" manual communication. William Holder, George Dalgarno, John Bulwer, and John Wallis disregarded oralism and the emphasis on speechreading and instead emphasized manual communication. In France, Michel Charles de l'Epeé received considerable acclaim for establishing a school for the deaf in Paris in the 1860s. His efforts brought together and secured the role of manual communication in institutions around the world (especially North America). During the same time period, however, Scotland and Germany's approach to deaf education emphasized speech and oralism (Winzer, 1998). John Amman, Jacob Periere, and Samual Heinicke publicly promoted the importance of speech and disregarded manual communication as a viable option. From this brief historical overview, it is important to recognize that the question of manual communication versus in oralism is not new. Since before Christ, people have pondered the origin of language. Various theories have been tried or tested on "those without language" including the deaf. Here, in A.D. 2000 the same questions remain. It is sufficient to say that the decisions about language and deafness should only be based on the needs of the individual, and not some nebulous and unresolved collective.

Not only has the controversy over educational interventions remain unresolved, services for the deaf have also experienced little significant change over the past several centuries. Mainstreaming and institutionalization continue to remain the two opposing "ideal" service models. Funding, location (urban vs. rural), and social status continue to remain critical factors in determining service availability. Religion, however, may have played a more prevalent role in the past as many schools were run by religious orders, and some are still closely related to these orders. Anne Quartararo (1995) author of "The Perils of Assimilation in Modern France: The Deaf Community, Social Status, and Educational Opportunity, 1815–1870" explains the prevailing issues and circumstances surrounding the educational practices in France. Not surprisingly, many of the same concerns continue to face today's educators. These issues include vocational training and employability of the deaf, mainstreaming and its effect on self-esteem, services for the "lower class" (now considered *marginalized populations*) and the role of speech in the language development of deaf children. Despite years of research, technological advances, and the introduction of the Deaf and hard of hearing perspective, the solutions to these issues remain elusive. Language development, early intervention strategies, and vocational training concerns continue to weigh heavily in the minds of the families of children with hearing loss.

Today, in modern day North America and other developed nations, services for children with hearing loss have become more individualized, emphasizing the needs of the family and the child as the most critical factor in determining service delivery. In Canada, and most other developed countries, residential institutions are slowly closing across the country, being replaced by community-based services. Individualized funding has given families more options when making their decisions about first language. To address the concerns of location and accessibility, the availability of early intervention programs has attempted to reach into the rural areas as well, ensuring most, if not all children have some type of family support. As well, formalized professions serving the deaf and hard of hearing population have evolved to include speech and language pathologists, hearing aid practitioners, audiologists, communication access real-time (CART) reporters, interpreters, early intervention specialists, and such. The list is extensive as well as exhaustive.

For a child with hearing impairments, technology and the need for a written language code become even more closely tied together as technology continues to have a profound effect on educational practices. What is the best way for the deaf and hard of hearing to benefit from these ongoing advances in technology? Live videophones, electronic mail, CART reporters, cochlear implants, high-tech hearing aids, and amplified telephones are only a few of the technological devices and services now available on the market. Many of these new devices emphasize the importance of having a written language (usually English) in order to make use of the potential benefit (i.e., captioning, distance education). Some inventions such as videoconferencing and video telephones continue to ensure that manual communication remains a viable option for those preferring to use some form of sign language, but, at present, such technology lags behind in its effectiveness. Other devices, such as advanced hearing aids and cochlear implants support the perspective that oralism remains the preferred method of communication and perhaps as well, language development. Technological advances in the past two decades have introduced tremendous change not only in educational practices (i.e., inclusive education and distance learning) but also in daily living (alarm clocks, visual fire alarms, etc.). Language development and the need/desire to benefit from technology are important considerations when choosing a first language.

OVERVIEW OF LANGUAGE AND COMMUNICATION

Before discussing language development and ethical implications, it is important to understand the relationship that exists between language and communication. While these words appear in everyday conversations, their technical definitions provide a unique insight necessary in understanding language development. For example, Owens (1996) explains that "language can be defined as a socially shared code or conventional system for representing concepts through the use of arbitrary symbols and rule-governed combinations of those symbols" (p. 8). With the understanding that language is simply a shared code, then "communication is the process participants use to exchange information of ideas, needs and desires. The process is an active one that involves encoding, transmitting, and decoding the intended message" (Owens, p. 9). Therefore, it can be said that communication and language are inherently locked together by the ability to use the shared code effectively.

Language itself is conveyed through a variety of modes (Owens, 1996). These modes include drawn symbols (used for reading and writing), through speech (verbal expression), and/or through manual communication of which the most advanced examples are some variant of sign language. Communication can also be broken into three different parts: paralinguistic (such as stress and emphasis, speed of delivery), metalinguistic (success of communication), and nonlinguistic (gestural, body posture, eye contact, etc.). Essentially, the intent to communicate with others and the ability to send or receive messages (using a combination of modes) that are meaningful are both necessary in creating effective communication. However, what happens when one individual is unable to create a message that is meaningful? That question is the foundation for the rest of the chapter.

ETHICAL FRAMEWORK

The decision-making process can be difficult for the family of a child with a hearing loss. Families are encouraged to make important decisions about language development as quickly as possible in order to ensure that any possible language-acquisition delay is minimized. Yet, often the information presented is inadequate and biased. Parents are presented specific information from well-meaning professionals such as cochlear implant teams or other professionals who have a well-defined and supported position, while perhaps what might be more helpful to the parents is additional information from support groups and adults who are willing to discuss their personal experiences as children with hearing losses. Although, technology has changed and advances have been made, families must remember that there is more to hearing loss than correcting hearing. The social, educational, and vocational implications of hearing loss require extended thought and discussion. "Fixing" the impairment is quite different from exploring the unique needs of a child with a hearing loss. It is clear why it is important for families to make these difficult decisions as soon as possible; however, the question of how to make these decisions is much more difficult. Choosing a first language is a complicated decision that involves a variety of factors. By creating a suitable framework, however, one might be able to make more sense of these factors and the roles that they play.

One potential framework is the process of understanding that the child has to be looked at in the context of self, family, and community. The second part of that process includes the addition of time lines. "Who are we now?" as compared to who we might become in 50 years' time. Both processes are essential to understanding the ethical implications of first language choice.

Example of Renn

Renn was a bright, happy, good-natured three-year-old when his parents discovered his "severe to profound" hearing loss. On the advice of the doctor, Mr. and Mrs. Hopowich contacted the local consultant to provide them with practical information regarding what steps to take to ensure language development. Being a strict believer in oral methods, the consultant put Renn's parents in touch with a speech pathologist/therapist who proceeded to work with both Renn and his parents.

Mrs. Hopowich was an elementary school teacher and Mr. Hopowich was a principal in the nearby junior high school. They recognized the importance of Renn learning language as a base for his future learning. Each day Mrs. Hopowich would sit with Renn for an hour and review all his exercises for speech training. She dutifully checked his hearing aids and F.M. system to be sure all was in working order. When Renn went to school the teachers, year after year, were informed of Renn's hearing loss and taught how to check his assistive listening equipment to ensure its proper performance. All was thought to be well when he learned to speak and to lip-read others' speech skillfully.

Unfortunately, it was not stressed to the teachers that when his or her back was turned Renn had no opportunity to see what he or she was saying. Renn was not provided with any extra help in the way of an oral interpreter, teacher's aid, or tutor and it was never considered that supplementary lecture/information notes might be helpful.

Each year Renn fell further behind. His speech abilities were very good, and when face to face his speech-reading skills were superb. In fact they were so good many people forgot he could not hear. No one had considered sensitivity training for the teachers or the students who shared his classes. Other children did not understand that he could not hear them yelling at him to come and join their play, nor that they would have to signal him visually to get his attention.

The acting-out behavior began in junior high school. By the time Renn was 20 and desperately wanting independence, he was angry, frustrated, lacked self-esteem, and had little sense of hope for his future. He had tried a few jobs, but his anger frequently prevented good working relationships with his peers. He trusted no one and thought the worst of people.

1. What should the consultant have advised?

2. Was the consultant wise to refer the parents only to a speech pathologist/therapist?

3. Why do you think Renn was acting out? Why did he become angry, frustrated, and lose self-esteem?

4. Without changing to a manual approach to language, how could things have been changed to reduce the frustration Renn experienced?

5. Would Renn benefit from learning sign language and involvement in the Deaf community?

To create a visual metaphor, think of the apocryphal stone being dropped in a pond. The ripples extend out past the initial place where the stone was dropped. These ripples are similar to the ones created by a new birth. The baby, a person in his or her own right becomes a child of one, or usually, two parents, perhaps a brother or sister, grandchild, niece or nephew, neighbor, potential customer for the local toy store, client for early intervention services, the list can go on. Using this concept, one is able to explore the context in which a child lives. The child is an individual who has been born into a family that has a value and belief system. This family belongs to an extended family that often shares a similar value and belief system. This extended family belongs to a community. The values and beliefs of the community can and will have a direct impact on the family. For example, the family's values and beliefs can be identified by the types of services available to the community members. Early intervention programs, local integrated day cares, and special education programs are all examples of the implementation of the values and beliefs of the community. With the understanding that a child with a hearing loss must survive within multiple value and belief systems, one can address the question "what happens when one individual is not able to create a message that is meaningful?"

Example of Ginny

Ginny developed meningitis at the age of two. Her parents were simple "country folk" who struggled to make ends meet. Upon discovering her profound hearing loss at age 3 the doctor suggested that the parents contact a special school for the deaf in a city 300 kilometers away. The school representative spent a number of hours with Mr. and Mrs. Podding, explaining the benefits of their daughter learning sign language and being in a school where deafness is well understood and educational accommodations are the norm. She would be with her peers, who share a common experience of the world, and communication would be rich.

It was decided Ginny would attend, but in order to do so she would have to live in a foster home. Mr. and Mrs. Podding had other children who had solid roots in their community. It would not be in their best interests to make a change in residence. They understood the long-term consequences of their little girl being isolated on the farm, and though they would miss their baby, it was "in her best interests." Within a few short months a wonderful foster home was found where a member of the family was an American Sign Language interpreter. All seemed well. Soon, however, Ginny's foster father was transferred to another city and Ginny would need to find a new home. Another family, the Coves, were quickly located but the advantage of having sign language in the home was lost. They were nice people, but too busy to take up sign language, and besides, they had other "handicapped" children living there. They were sure Ginny would adapt well. Ginny stayed with them year after year and went to her own family's home for special holidays and long weekends.

As a youngster Ginny participated in all the family outings, games, and activities, but as a teenager she grew tired of not having any communication at home. She was lonely at home and longed to be with her friends where she could understand and be understood readily. There were often misunderstandings: what time to be home, where she was going, what she would be doing, who she would be with. There were many times she was given consequences for her behavior but did not understand what she had done wrong. She moped around the house waiting for the next moment she would be with her friends. Holidays and long weekends were different. Going to her birth parents' home was boring. No one talked to her. They would smile, nod their heads, point and gesture, but real communication—it was not!

From Mr. and Mrs. Cove's perspective, Ginny was willful, determined, stubborn, temperamental, and hard to handle. She refused to sit down and do her homework. She would not sit down with the family to watch TV. She would not take part in any of the family discussions, even when the outcome would affect her. They could not understand what her problem was; and it was "sad that she would not even try to lip-read or speak!" The other "handicapped kids were much easier to handle."

At the age of 18, Ginny, in her last year at the school for the deaf, began to think of employment and independence. She had worked part-time at a few places, but it was always the same: no one there to talk to. She did not look forward to future employment and only wanted to be with her friends. Unlike other Deaf people, she decided she would just apply for social services and that way she would not have to put up with the boring life of no one to communicate with. She could live on her own and spend time with her friends whenever she wanted.

1. What other options could the parents have explored?
2. Why did Ginny become so "difficult"?
3. How could the Cove family have avoided the misunderstandings?
4. Is isolation an absolute for a deaf child in a rural community?
5. Would Ginny have been better to stay at home and be educated at the local community school?
6. Were the Poddings well advised to think the only option was the school for the deaf?

This is where language and communication become critical considerations. What is the language of the family? What language codes are available in the community? In many developed countries, where technology is quite advanced, parents have a multitude of choices in choosing a language code. Examples include but are not limited to Auditory-Verbal, Auditory-Oral, Cued Speech, Total Communication, and a variety of Manually Coded English systems. These alternative language codes each have advantages and disadvantages. (For specific information about these approaches see the Web sites found in libraries or on the Internet, a selection of which is given at the end of this chapter in the addendum.) Often the information available can be overwhelming and conflicting. Parents and professionals alike can become disillusioned with the controversy and confusion surrounding language development. From a historical perspective, however, the question of best practices in language development remains unsolved. This is an important point. The lack of success in determining best practices of language development means that the family becomes the "expert" on determining the needs of their child. The family knows and understands best what the home environment of the child is and how communication and language exist in the home. Parents can be encouraged to identify their strengths as a family unit, and how these strengths can be enhanced in order for the child to succeed.

An example of this could be the decision for the family to learn ASL so that the child would benefit from having a visual language (e.g., Casey at the beginning of the chapter). Family members could learn ASL at the local education center and become involved with the Deaf community. This would ensure that the child was exposed to Deaf language role models and assist the family in exploring the social and emotional developmental aspects of hearing loss. One of the advantages of this preferred communication method is the perspective that the child would learn the visual language code considered "ideal" by the Deaf community. Another important advantage is that the visual language code would take advantage of the child's ability to process language cognitively without impaired perceptual differences. In addition, the use of ASL would ensure that there was a consistent language code among family members at home and between home and school, allowing communication to occur freely between all. This would be in contrast to the child feeling "left out" of verbal conversations in which the child could not "hear."

While there are numerous advantages to implementing a manual language code in the family home, it is also necessary to identify the disadvantages. Remember that learning a new language is difficult for any adult, and it is unlikely that fluency could be obtained in a short time. Time, money, and dedication are more examples of important factors that could affect the efforts of committed parents. Other children in the home, support from the extended family, and community intervention services are examples of extraneous variables that can positively or negatively influence the success of this effort. In Casey's situation in the opening case study, the parents have chosen the "ideal" solution that would ensure that the child learned a first language that was natural to him or her and would allow for future membership in the culturally Deaf community. Still, limitations of the family and community systems could negatively affect the language development, resulting in confusion and chaos in the child's perception of the world. This is not to say that a family effort to learn ASL is wrong. Instead, the family should seek to ensure that supports are in place in order to maximize success and minimize harm of any approach they have chosen. Other language codes as listed earlier can also be demanding and require intense family and community commitment. It is the ability of the family to adapt and to implement communication and language learning strategies that become essential considerations when choosing a first language.

Example of Sandra

Sandra was born deaf and was discovered at an early age. The local consultant led her mother, Mrs. Gagne, through a program that professed miracles for deaf children learning English. The consultant had stressed to Mrs. Gagne that if she was not strong enough to fight battles with the school board little Sandra would be "like the rest of the Deaf community—able to read and write at the equivalent of grade three as an adult." Mrs. Gagne was adamant Sandra would learn English and be competent in school. She had been a nurse, but before her first child was born she returned to school to get her teaching degree. Sandra was enrolled in a special, local play school for Signing Exact English (SEE-II), by the age of 2 years. Mr. and Mrs. Gagne actively took part in learning SEE-II at night and hired a tutor to practice with on the evenings they were not in class. The tutor was also hired to work with Sandra's siblings, Randy and David, to teach them SEE-II. As Sandra was growing up Mrs. Gagne worked hard with her. She gave her speech lessons, as she was instructed to do, and read with her often. The whole family, siblings included, signed when they talked, so Sandra would be included as an equal in the home. The family had been told that if Sandra were ever exposed to American Sign Language (ASL), her ability to learn English would be diminished. Mr. and Mrs. Gagne outlawed the use of any ASL signs or homemade signs. If one of them did not know a sign for a word, or forgot the sign, he or she would have to fingerspell. They felt it would be good practice for the other children too, in that they would benefit from the spelling practice.

As Sandra was growing up she had her family around her all the time. Her siblings went to the same school: one sibling two years ahead and the other a year behind. A SEE-II transliterator was provided for her, right at the beginning of grade one. Her situation was perfect for good communication, and her marks showed it. Her marks were better than many of the hearing students and she excelled in all she did. Her English was exemplary.

Unfortunately, the intense focus on Sandra was causing Randy and David to become resentful, and they felt like they did not have the love and attention of their parents. Everything was for Sandra. They began to withdraw from family gatherings, tease Sandra and say mean things to her. They did not associate with other kids in school because there were always a million questions about Sandra and their mom. The kids started to avoid Sandra in junior high, and by high school none of the kids at school wanted to spend time with her. Everywhere she went her mother was there. After awhile, the school was uncomfortable hiring staff to work with Sandra because if the slightest thing was not to Sandra's liking, her mother would storm in to make sure everything was put the way she wanted it. She was a straightforward, blunt type of woman. Sandra herself began to see what power her mother had and began to play games with the transliterators. "I can get you fired you know? All I have to do is tell my mom I don't like you and you're a goner."

1. Did this family work toward keeping the family together?
2. Was the decision to choose Signing Exact English (SEE-II) a good one?
3. If the language choice was not the problem here, what was?
4. Is there anything that a professional could have done early on to help the family avoid this kind of unpleasant situation?
5. Could a professional help the family resolve this situation now it has developed so negatively?

Exploring the child's role in the family and in the community is an essential part of the decision-making process. The child has the right to belong to the family, and not feel left out due to language and communication barriers. Full participation in family and community activities is part of every child's natural development. Maximizing the individual strengths of the child is an important part of choosing a first language. There are a variety of questions that parents might ask themselves about their child and their family home. What communication style does the child appear to feel most comfortable using? Which approach seems least intrusive to the child and the family home? Are there any additional problems that might prevent the successful use of a specific communication style (e.g., clef palate, cerebral palsy, vision impairment)?

Community supports include a variety of informal and formal systems that lead to the language development of a child diagnosed with a hearing loss. Parents must be encouraged to question the type and availability of supports in their area. For example, these supports can be influenced by location (urban vs. rural), socioeconomic status of the community, availability of trained professionals, and family participation in community activities (i.e., church, local parent group). If a child accesses the nearest urban center for a cochlear implant, will the follow-up services be adequate? Will the child and community supports (i.e., early intervention specialist, educators) receive sufficient assistance to maximize the benefit of the implant? If the family pursues a visual language code, are there sign language interpreters available in the local school system? Will the educators be able to support the needs of the child in the school system, or will the child need to attend a residential school? Understanding the resources available in the family's local community is an important part of the decision-making process about a child's first language.

Example of Bobby and Alisa

Bobby and Alisa were born two years apart, both of them later diagnosed with severe hearing losses. Mr. and Mrs. Rutamin lived in a small town in northern Manitoba and felt it was important to keep their children at home, where they could be well cared for by the family. The itinerant teacher made frequent visits to the school and family to ensure all was going well. Speech and language exercises were given to Mrs. Rutamin to practice with the children and the itinerant teacher taught sign language to Mr. and Mrs. Rutamin. A sign club was set up at the school for Bobby and Alisa's peers to learn to communicate with them. Teacher's aids were hired to work with both of them and, for the first few years, things went well. The children did well in school and they got along with their peers.

However, as they grew older, each in turn began to struggle in school. As Bobby began junior high school his grades dropped drastically. He still had lots of friends and was very popular, but he was not able to grasp some of the key courses at school. He did fine in math, art, and

*physical education but social studies, science, and English began to lag.
Two years later a similar situation started to develop for Alisa.*

*During an interview with the teachers, teacher's aids, and parents it
became apparent that the teacher's aids had taken sign language classes
specifically to learn to work with Bobby and Alisa when they first entered
the school system. Both Mrs. Roberts and Miss Jelowski had taken levels
one, two, and three. Levels one and two had been offered on weekends at a
major city two-and-a-half hours from home, but when they took level three
they had to travel there after school, and then back again late at night to be
ready for work the next morning. They did not go on to level four because
they felt that with their sign language dictionary and the training they had
received, they had enough skills to work with the children at the elementary
level. Now, however, in junior high school, it was getting tougher.*

1. Why were the children's grades dropping?
2. What options might be available to the family?
3. What options might be available to the school?
4. What would you recommend for Bobby and Alisa to improve their
   performance in school?
5. What other options could the school board have followed?

Not only is it necessary to determine what the community resources are, but
also to understand how the family defines their child's hearing loss, because this
will directly influence their perception of community resources. For example, if
the family unit is committed to implementing ASL as their primary language
code, they would be more likely to seek out Deaf associations and educational
programs that support the teaching of ASL. If, however, a family were inclined to
pursue a cochlear implant or other technological aids, the services of an audiologist would be more beneficial.

REFLECTIONS

In the opening illustrative case study, the influence of earlier decisions on the educational process and of the emotional well-being of Casey, are well documented. Casey
has failed to reach his potential in the academic core areas because of a number of
deliberate or tangential decisions that have left him poorly prepared for schoolwork
in these subjects. He is falling behind, and catching up will be extremely difficult if
not impossible. Equally of concern is that he is also showing early signs of what
could become major behavioral problems in school and mental health problems in
adult life. His lack of a "natural" language, of whatever form, is a classic example of
Kanapell's axiom: "To deny my language is to deny myself." To not have a language
is, to not only deny my person, but an explicit example of the Whorfian[1] hypothesis.
Our language shapes us, and who we are shapes our language.

Yet, how many professionals have a perspective of the whole life span of our students or clients? Do we know the experiences of Deaf or hard of hearing adults? Equally, do professionals working with adults know of the demands, challenges, and skills required to teach young deaf or hard of hearing children? Ethically, we have no right to make pronouncements on matters of which we have no direct professional experience. To have been a child in school may give us valuable insights and some empathy. However, only by teaching or working professionally in a preschool program are we able to gain the knowledge and understanding of the practice in respect of the needs of Deaf and hard of hearing students in such programs. Each of us brings our own personal perspective to our professional judgments. Most of us have much to learn from qualitative research paradigms and their focus on a declaration of personal bias. Perhaps all of us need to examine our personal biases before we enter into any pronouncements about programs: whether for individual students, children or adults, or for the collective. In our opinion such a procedure would dramatically reduce the schisms that litter our professional practice like the tragic battlefields of so many human conflicts. Such schisms are often an example of man's inhumanity to man.

So, could Casey's life have been different, or could it become different? In the past—yes. The parents could have been given information not dogma. They could have been supported in the genesis of their efforts to provide help and support for their child. They could have been respected for what they did, rather than attacked for what they were unable to do because of the unrealistic expectations placed on them by professionals.[2]

The effects of exposure to such a variety of language codes could and should have been recognized by professionals, as should the high level of Casey's cognitive abilities. There should have been a recognition of the "blaming the victim" syndrome, whereby Casey was held to be responsible for his own failure. This recognition will become even more important to his "behavioral" difficulties if they continue to increase. The older he is and the less his problems are defined as educational, the more he will be pathologized. When this happens, the self-fulfilling prophecy will be fulfilled and the professionals will hide behind the smoke screen of jargon and rhetoric. The poor parents, after all, are the ultimate culprits, and our Old Testament morality will prevail: the "defective" child is a visitation of God's wrath for the sins of the mother (and occasionally the father). Who are we to subvert the will of God by succeeding where he/she has failed?

And what of the future? Casey is 10 years old. If the foundations of language are not laid by this age or shortly thereafter, the prognosis is not good. Will he become a Gemini child trapped in a poverty of environment to emerge into a plethora of well-meaning professionals whose response to failure is to return the problem to the institution and system from which it had the tenacity to emerge? Probably, but not with certainty. He may be lucky. He may meet a teacher who understands that if you do not have language, you can only achieve it through Bruner's "playful ambience."[3] Whether the Barry's original "five slates" method or Blackwell's five sentence patterns, we do not learn language through structure.

No! We learn the structure (of language) through the language. Or as David Wood put it: the problem of schools for deaf children is that they operate on the premise that children have developed language before they enter school. (For an extended discussion see Wood, Wood, Griffiths, & Howarth; 1986.) When, like Casey, children have not developed language before they enter schools, educational philosophy and practice whether in regular, special, or "deaf" education, is ill prepared to deal with them. There are some powerful and notable exceptions, however, some of whom have written other chapters in this book. But they are the exception that proves the rule.

REFERENCES

Deacon, J. J. (1974). *Tongue tied.* New York: Scribner.

Harris, G. A. (1983). *Broken ears, wounded heart.* Washington, DC: Gallaudet College Press.

Owens, R. E. Jr. (1996). *Language development: An introduction* (4th ed.). Needham Heights, MA: Allyn & Bacon.

Quartararo, A. T., (1995). The perils of assimilation in modern France: The deaf community, social status, and education opportunity, 1815–1870. *Journal of Social History, 29*(1), 5–25.

Winzer, M. A., (1998). A tale often told: The early progression of special education. *Remedial and Special Education, 19*(4), 212–219.

Wood, D., Wood, H., Griffiths, A., & Howarth, I. (1986). *Teaching and talking with deaf children.* Chichester: John Wiley and Sons.

FURTHER READINGS

Calderon, R., & Green, M. T. (1999). Stress and coping in hearing mothers of children with hearing loss: Factors affecting mother and child adjustment. *American Annals of the Deaf, 44*(2), 7–17.

Grosjean, F. (1992). The bilingual and the bicultural person in the hearing and in the Deaf world. *Sign Language Studies, 77,* 307–320.

Henderson, D., & Hendershott, A. (1991). ASL and the family system. *American Annals of the Deaf, 136,* 325–329.

Luetke-Stahlman, B. (1992). Comparing four input models of parental questions to hearing and deaf preschoolers. *ACEHI Journal, 18*(2/3), 93–101.

Vis Dubé, R. (1995). Creating a bilingual environment for children who are deaf. *ACEHI Journal, 21*(1), 62–68.

APPENDIX

Important or Main Points

- Language development has been pondered and examined by many of the great philosophers of the world.

  We know, therefore, that the concept of language development is complex, and with many questions and few answers. Choosing a first language and an appropriate language development model is not to be taken lightly or based on happenstance. The question requires research, reflection, and introspective thinking.

- The family is the expert on the child.

    This is the most important concept of the ethical framework. The family knows (or can be coached to recognize) its strengths and its ability to adapt and make changes. Professional consultation is an important part of obtaining the information necessary to make an informed decision; however, the family should have the first and last say on the developmental approach.

- Recognize and encourage the child's right to belong and participate in the community.

    Remember that the child will need to socialize with others in the community, outside the family unit. As the child matures, he or she will move away from the family unit and a become contributing member to society. To do so, the child must have a solid language base and a communication method that will allow for and encourage full participation.

- Everyone brings their own personal perspective to their professional judgments.

    Most professionals have much to learn from qualitative research paradigms and their focus on a declaration of personal bias. Perhaps everyone needs to examine their personal biases before they enter into any pronouncements about programs: whether for individual students, children or adults, or for the collective.

Follow-up References or Suggestions

Internet

The following is a brief list of some of the multitude of Web sites providing information about hearing loss and children (including some on language development). The descriptive remarks in quotations mean that the information was taken directly from the Web site itself. Many of the Web sites listed here include a variety of links that will provide additional information about hearing loss with children. When accessing these sites, please remember that there is no regulating body on the Internet and that the information obtained should be discussed with your family support team.

- http://www.audiologynet.com/

    "AudiologyNet is an audiology and hearing healthcare informational Web site for a large population. It is dedicated to providing Web site links in audiology for patients, family members, students, and healthcare providers."

- http://www.voicefordeafkids.com/

    "To ensure that all Hearing Impaired Children have the right to develop their ability to listen and speak and have access to services which will enable them to listen and speak." (Site provides information about Auditory Verbal Therapy, and includes support information for parents.)

- http://www.auditory-verbal.org/
  "Auditory-Verbal International, Inc (AVI) is a private nonprofit international membership organization whose principal objective is to promote listening and speaking as a way of life for children who are deaf or hard of hearing."

- http://www.agbell.org/publications/periodicals.html
  "AG Bell focuses specifically on children with hearing loss, providing ongoing support and advocacy for parents, professionals and other interested parties." (Provides a variety of useful information for families and professionals.)

- http://www.hipmag.org/
  A fun magazine specifically for kids with hearing loss.

- http://faculty.washington.edu/chudler/bigear.html
  A fun Web site that explains "The Ear," using plenty of visual pictures.

- http://dww.deafworldweb.org/pub/b/bi.rights99.html
  A Web site that contains a position paper entitled "The right of deaf child to grow bilingual."

- http://www.augie.edu/perry/ar/ar.htm
  A Web site that provides extensive information and links about audiological rehabilitation (including links about cochlear implants).

- http://www.oraldeafed.org/
  "Here, you will find specific information about these schools and their programs and services, and other information on oral deaf education in our Library."

- http://www2.pair.com/options/info.htm
  Gives a brief explanation of Auditory-Verbal, Auditory-Oral, Cued Speech, Total Communication, and American Sign Language approaches along with the related links to other organizations.

- http://www.isl.net/~cuedspmn/Welcome.html
  Provides in-depth information on cued speech including a resource list for those searching for more specific definitions and ideas.

Books

This is a limited list of books that have provided unique insight into deafness and language development.

- Lane, H., (1992). *The mask of benevolence: Disabling the Deaf community.* Toronto: Random House of Canada.
  An excellent book describing the history of the deaf. Lane discusses the historical role of the "experts and professions" in the evolution of deafness. This text provides a powerful and moving position on the role of manual

communication in the lives of the deaf. It is, however, emotional and somewhat biased in its presentation. Therefore, its objectivity can sometimes be questioned.

- Owens, R. E. Jr. (2000). *Language development: An introduction* (5th ed.). S. D. Dragin. (Ed.) Boston: Allyn & Bacon.
  This is an excellent introductory text that thoroughly explains the models of language development as well as the developmental stages. It is a textbook used in many university courses on language development.

- Sacks, O. (1989). *Seeing voices.* Berkeley and Los Angeles, CA: University of California press
  Oliver Sacks provides a unique look at deafness and sign language. His historical research as well as his personal reflections and experiences provide a dynamic and interesting read.

Ethical Questions for Consideration

- Is the predictive ability of deafness experts good enough to identify those deaf children and families who have the necessary abilities and conditions to be successful with learning either an aural-oral or a visual-manual language?
- What are the implications of choosing a mother tongue for a child that is different from the parents or the other family members? (Consider the situation of second language using parents.)
- Although there appears to be an elegant compromise between visual-manual and auditory-oral realities and outcomes when a signed oral-language is selected for a deaf child, how does one cope with the reality that the facility of most parents and educators with that language is less than adequate?
- Although choosing a mother tongue or first language may be seen as the first decision that arises, it usually isn't done unless the method of language learning and the use of assessment and amplification is considered simultaneously. Are parents simply overwhelmed by this mass of information and would better-timed delivery systems make for better decisions?
- Although most people consider the polar options readily—that being, visual-manual for the deaf-of-deaf, and auditory-oral for the deaf-of-hearing—there is still a consideration "middle ground" where people take a "central" position of using a sign system reflective of an oral language. Can even the developed nations support all of the educational variations these choices entail?
- The choice of language is almost always reflected in the reality that 9 or 10 deaf children have hearing parents. Thus is it true that the minority, the deaf parents with deaf children, are like hearing parents of hearing children, and do not usually need to ponder the language decision extensively?

NOTES

[1] Whorf's theory of linguistic determination states that thought is determined by language. Therefore users of different languages have different experiences and understanding of their world. For example, is a Deaf person's perception of God shaped by the fact that the understanding of omnipotence cannot be the same for Deaf children? Does their God "speak to them in voices" which they hear or "sign to them in signs that they can see"? If so, how can they conceive of God's presence in the absence of a visual image?

[2] Those who doubt the validity of such a claim should read *Broken Ears, Wounded Hearts* by George A. Harris published in 1983 or from another area of disability the book *Tongue Tied* by Joseph John (Joey) Deacon of 1974.

[3] Bruner's theory is that children only learn language through "playful" interaction with parents or surrogate parents. They cannot be taught language through formal instruction. David Wood extends this concept to explain that schools are poor places to teach early language. The assumption, for both hearing and deaf students, is that children come to schools with an already developed language. Many teachers of Deaf and hard of hearing students have this implicit assumption in the way they relate to their students, even though they will explicitly reject the hypothesis, and would seem to agree with Bruner and Wood.

5

ETHICS OF ASSESSMENT

ELEANOR STEWART AND KATHRYN RITTER[1]

AUTHOR INTRODUCTION—
ELEANOR STEWART[2]

After spending many years as a speech-language pathologist pondering questions about how we practice and what relationship we ought to have with families we serve and the institutions we work in (or around), I chose to pursue a course of study in the area of bioethics.

Growing up in a family with a member who is severely hearing impaired has had an impact on my clinical work and revealed to me questions about legitimate knowledge, power, and the tension between subjectivity and objectivity in clinical decision making.

While I remain committed to the liberal ideal of individual choice, I am cognizant, as a clinician and as a parent, of the very real barriers to the exercise of choice in health care. In my studies, I set out to learn about how choice is presented and acted upon. This exploration brought me to the broader issues of social justice: race, class, gender, and (dis)ability. And the context in which these issues are played out: liberal democracy.

In my clinical years, I worked with families of infants, toddlers, and preschoolers with a variety of communication disorders including deafness. Many of the children I worked with had severe physical limitations as well. They were graduates of neonatal intensive care and had survived at immense cost.

I have an undergraduate degree in psychology from Dalhousie University, a master's in speech-language pathology from the University of Kansas, and am completing a doctorate in rehabilitation science with a specialization in bioethics at the University of Alberta. I served on both the clinical and research ethics committees of the Glenrose Rehabilitation Hospital. I have also served on the ethics committee of the Canadian Association of Speech-Language Pathologists and Audiologists and continue to serve as Chair of the Ethics Committee of the Speech-Language-Hearing Association of Alberta.

AUTHOR INTRODUCTION—KATHRYN RITTER[3]

I have been a teacher of the deaf in Language and Speech Services for the Hearing Impaired at Glenrose Rehabilitation Hospital in Edmonton since 1975. During that time, the primary goal of my work has been to enable families to support their children's communication and learning in optimal ways. It has always been clear to me that families exert the greatest influence on their child's overall ability to lead happy, productive lives. As a clinician committed to family centered practice, I am compelled to accept and support the family's decisions about what is best for their child and their family. This is not always easy. It is challenging to find ways to support families when their concept of what is best for their child differs substantially from one's own. That challenge is the source of a great deal of learning and personal growth.

I hold a BSc in Speech-Language Pathology from Southwest Missouri State University, a MSc in Education of the Deaf from the University of Kansas, and a PhD in Special Education from the University of Alberta. I hold certifications from the Association of Canadian Educators of the Deaf and Hard of Hearing, the Council on Education of the Deaf in the United States, and Auditory-Verbal International. Most of the national and international conference presentations that I have done, as well as published articles in Canada and the United States, have been concerned with issues of families rights to be supported in their choices and in the creation of effective collaborations between families and professionals.

A CASE TO CONSIDER[4]

Sara's Mother: My daughter, Sara, had meningitis when she was 18 months old. Our family lived in a small community in northern Canada. Sara had been emergency evacuated to the nearest large city, 800 kilometers away, for medical treatment and rehabilitation. I flew down with her, trying to keep my fear in check so that I could comfort Sara. I left behind our four older children. I left behind my husband—his support, his faith, his strength so needed now and so far away. I remember the steady sound of engines. I remember praying.

Some things about that time are very clear—others are a blur. Sara was ill and in pain for a long time. We almost lost her, but her spirit is strong. I knew that she would survive before the doctors told me so. Just as I was allowing myself to feel relief, her doctor asked for permission to have an audiologist perform an Auditory Brainstem test to find out if her hearing had been affected. She told me that meningitis sometimes caused hearing loss. She asked for permission to sedate Sara for the test. Sara had just undergone an intense struggle for her life. I was not prepared to have her sedated. I was willing to accept a hearing loss as the price of her survival and felt no urgency to confirm it. My stronger urge was to protect Sara from more invasive medical procedures. I wanted her to have time to recover from her ordeal, a chance for her spirit to heal her body as fully as possible. I would do what was necessary for her hearing when I was sure she'd had enough time to do that. I wanted to take her home, to celebrate her healing with my husband and her brothers and sisters.

Sara's Audiologist: Sara is a beautiful, intelligent child. I met her during a routine follow-up appointment that her doctor arranged after she had recovered from meningitis. Her mother seemed defensive and very protective.

I always struggle with this. Parents are often not ready to be confronted with their child's hearing status after they survive a serious illness. They simply can't deal with the thought that the ordeal isn't over. If you are committed, as I am, to family-centered treatment, you are constantly torn between the need to assert your expertise in what you believe are the child's best interests, and the need to respect the parents' process and priorities. This mother had refused to have her child sedated for an ABR. I understood her resistance to sedating her daughter after such an ordeal, but a Brainstem test is the best way to be certain of the child's hearing status at Sara's age. And if we can get a fairly accurate assessment, we can get the early start on amplification that we know is so important for the development of listening and speech skills.

Sara's mother did let us try Visual Reinforcement Audiometry. It doesn't require sedation, and Sara seemed so bright that I thought we might be able to get a reasonable assessment with her just listening in the sound suite and reinforcing her responses to sound with lights. I asked Sara's mother if she thought Sara could hear, but she said Sara's ability to hear was not her primary concern at this point. She felt that it was much more important to reunite Sara with her family. She was only seeing me today because her doctor didn't want to discharge Sara from the hospital until her hearing had been tested. I wish I could make this easier.

Sara's complete lack of response in the sound suite made me certain that she had a severe to profound hearing loss. I think her mother realized that Sara's hearing was quite damaged as well. She was very quiet as I offered her the Brainstem test again before she went back up North. I remember thinking, "Please let us do this! It could make such a big difference to Sara!" She was adamant, though. She wanted home, and family, and normalcy. She wasn't ready to be convinced by some objective test that Sara's life, and therefore her family's life, was changed forever. I knew it was time to let go, but knowing the likely consequences of delay makes that terribly difficult.

Sara's Mother: Sara is deaf. I felt fairly certain of it before we went into the soundproof room. As I sat there, holding Sara and watching for a response as the sound got louder and louder, I felt a sure, sorrowful confirmation enter my heart. My baby was deaf—but she was alive, and still had the same beautiful smile and quick intelligence that she had always had. I needed to get her home. I needed to be home, in the shelter and solace of my husband and my children's love. We had been away, in the city, for almost a month. Sara's healing would be completed in the clean, cold air and open skies of our Northern home. We would decide together what to do next. We would listen to our daughter, try to understand what she needed, and then we would do what we believed needed to be done about her hearing.

Sara's Audiologist: Sara's parents are, at last, able to address Sara's hearing loss. We've lost the last six months, time when Sara might have been hearing, or during which we might have become sure enough of how she would do with hearing aids to know whether they would even help her. She's lost most of the speech she had, and it's obvious that she's frustrated about communication. The Auditory Brainstem test confirmed a profound, bilateral hearing loss—her brain waves showed no responses to the limits of the equipment. There was no response on her Otoacoustic Emission test either, so we have additional confirmation that her cochleas are badly damaged.

We've arranged a trial fitting of hearing aids, and a meeting with our team's speech-language pathologist and teacher of the deaf to assess Sara's communication skills and give her parents some suggestions about how to work with Sara. I can see that Sara's parents' priorities and those to which I am committed are at odds. All of these people barging into their lives, providing information that they are sure Sara's parents need—I can see that the kind of structured, intensive work on communication that we believe will benefit Sara is not consistent with her parents' way of interacting with their children. They are a quiet, joyful, intelligent couple. It is not in their nature to focus on what is wrong, and yet, that's our job—to address what's wrong.

Sara is so bright that she would be a good candidate for a cochlear implant, but her parents have to follow through with hearing aids first. And the longer we wait, the more likely it is that Sara's cochlea's will ossify—fill up with bone, due to the meningitis. That might make an implant impossible. I've tried to help them understand the importance of time, but I get the feeling that they're not committed to the hearing aids, let alone the possibility of cochlear implantation.

Sara's Mother: Sara has grown well and strong. It has been a great joy for us to watch her return to herself again. Communication has become a struggle though. We use lots of gestures and pantomime, and Sara has become a master at communicating this way, but more and more it is clear that this won't be enough. Because of this, we decided to return to the audiologist, get the recommended testing done and see if they could help Sara communicate more easily with us. I hated having her sedated, taking her consciousness away so that the audiologist could attach electrodes to her head with an adhesive. Then sitting for a time that seemed like forever, listening to clicks and watching screens displaying the activity of her brain that was uninterpretable to me. Then the results, unsurprising by now—a profound hearing loss. Recommendations about hearing aids. A meeting with two other professionals who tell me that Sara's speech and language are now significantly delayed. Discussions about methods of communication—sign language, oral, auditory-verbal. The possibility that hearing aids will make little or no difference.

The audiologist squirts a soft, gooey substance into Sara's ear—earmold impressions. Sara squirms and makes a face, but tolerates it. During the two weeks that we wait for the earmolds to come in, I have a series of appointments with a speech pathologist and a teacher of the deaf to explore communication methods. Sara's hearing loss is so profound that it's likely that sign language will be her most fluent communication method. I read books from the parent library. I buy a sign language dictionary. I start practicing with Sara, and she begins to imitate almost immediately.

Finally, the earmolds arrive, and we try her new hearing aids. Putting these things in my perfect child's ears feels wrong. She doesn't like wearing them, and I don't see any difference in her ability to hear with them. Nevertheless, I believe we have to try. Sara needs a chance to discover how she will be most comfortable with herself and with us. It's our job to introduce her to her possible choices. The audiologist explained to me that young children with profound hearing losses often require some time before they respond to hearing aids because, even with the aids, the sounds they hear are very soft and might not catch their attention.

Sara's Audiologist: Sara has had her hearing aids for three months, but gets very little benefit from them. I am now certain that she would do much better with a cochlear implant. Her parents, after their long initial delay, surprised me with their commitment to keeping the aids on Sara. They have also done a good job introducing her to signed communication—Sara now uses about 50 signs and is starting to combine signs into short phrases. Her voice quality and use of voice in general have deteriorated quite a lot since the last time I saw her. I started discussing the possibility of a cochlear implant with Sara's mother on their last visit.

Sara's Mother: The audiologist has spoken to me about a cochlear implant for Sara. She explained the surgery, the required CT scan, the additional hearing testing, the possible benefits. She offered no guarantees that Sara would be able to understand and talk well enough to be easily understood, but offered hope of the possibility in the examples of many other children who had developed this ability as a result of the implant. The ability to speak and to understand speech would give Sara much greater freedom than sign language would allow her, although she loves to sign and is good at it. But the idea of introducing something foreign into her body goes strongly against our traditional beliefs about maintaining the integrity of our bodies so that the union of mind, body, and spirit is not endangered. The audiologist seems certain that a cochlear implant is the best option for Sara, will offer her the widest array of choices in the future. This decision will be the most difficult one we have had to make so far.

We understand that if we wait, this might not be an option for Sara in the future. It might not even be an option now—it would take another sedation and a CT scan to see if her cochleas are still open or if they have filled up with bone. Is the possibility of widening the circle of people with whom she might be able to communicate worth the intrusion into her life, her body, our lives? If we lived in the city it might be different, but no one outside of our family here has any signing ability. We feel sometimes as if she is starved for stimulation, interaction, communication. What will it be like to grow up with that kind of isolation? Will she be angry with us for not doing it? Will she be angry with us for doing it? The consequences either way seem too large.

ETHICS OF ASSESSMENT: AN INTRODUCTION

Audiological assessment of hearing loss in the pediatric population involves a significant investment of time, technical resources, intellectual and emotional resources. In infancy, it involves at least two professionals, and often as many as four. In locations where universal infant screening takes place, the initial screening is often done by a technician. Confirmation of the screen results frequently involves the family physician, an audiologist, and an Ear Nose and Throat Specialist. All of these resources are engaged before the habilitation or rehabilitation process (including fitting of amplification) is initiated, and yet this aspect of hearing loss has received little ethical examination. Certainly, individuals engaged in the process are bound by their profession's code of ethics, but ethical issues arising from the effect of the assessment process on children and families merit discussion.

The pediatric assessment process is often extremely stressful for parents. Although some Deaf parents may welcome a diagnosis of deafness, most hearing parents experience a great deal of anxiety during the process, which might take place over days, weeks, or even months depending on access to professionals and technical resources. The vast majority of parents who receive a diagnosis of hearing loss for their child are hearing people (90 to 95 %). Many have had no experience with hearing loss, and receive a positive diagnosis with shock, fear, disbelief, or grief. Because some of our readers will be familiar with the audiological assessment process and some will not, a description of the process as it typically occurs is provided in an Appendix to ensure that our readers have a shared context for our discussion.

Cochlear Implantation

Depending on the results of the basic audiological assessment process, and a trial period of appropriate amplification, cochlear implantation may be presented to families as an option for their child. Cochlear implantation, as many readers are aware, requires a surgical procedure to implant an array of electrodes in the child's cochlea that provide electrical stimulation to the auditory nerve, bypassing the damaged hair cells in the cochlea that are the cause of most sensorineural hearing losses. The surgery itself takes approximately 3 hours, and usually requires one or two full days in the hospital to monitor recovery prior to discharge. After four weeks to allow for healing, the process of activating and programming the implant takes place.

Although this procedure does not restore normal hearing, it provides many recipients with sound perception that allows them to develop comprehension and use of spoken language, particularly if done at age 2 or younger (Geers & Moog, 1994). Reflecting the rapidly accumulating evidence of the efficacy of cochlear implantation (see Waltzman & Cohen, 2000, for the most recent and comprehensive review of the process) the criteria for candidacy is expanding to include severe as well as profound hearing losses, and to include a wider range of people in terms of age and functional status.

Assessment for cochlear implantation represents a significant expansion of the initial process (Hellman et al., 1991). Depending on the age of the child, a variety of speech perception tests are done, as well as psychological assessment in many centers to assist clinicians in counseling parents as accurately as possible regarding expected outcomes. Parent questionnaires explore the child's functional use of hearing and parental expectations. In some centers this is complemented by a social work assessment to ensure that parental expectations are appropriate. Medical candidacy is confirmed through CT scan or MRI, both of which require sedation for children. The family's ability and willingness to access these services and to participate actively in the process are necessary.

There is a wealth of literature supporting the benefits of early identification and of early, optimal amplification. (See Yoshinaga-Itano, 1998 and Yoshinaga-Itano, Sedely, Coulter, & Mehl, 1998 for an extended discussion and reference list.) Some, however, feel that the process is too invasive and prolonged despite reported benefits, or, in a cultural view of deafness, inappropriate as an effort to "fix" deafness. Frequently cited ethical questions about cochlear implantation concern informed consent and resource allocation. A list of other possible ethical questions arising from the assessment process can be found at the conclusion of this chapter.

Readers may have expected us to focus on cochlear implantation as the central issue of this chapter, but we believe that this would be inappropriate. This process and the many ethical questions arising from it have been the subject of a great deal of treatment in the scholarly and popular press. Interested readers are invited to sample this literature in the suggested reading list at the end of this chapter.

Communication Assessment

Audiological evaluation is only one aspect of the assessment process that children with hearing loss and their families typically undergo. The assessment of the child's communication skill becomes an ongoing part of the child's life from the day the hearing loss is identified. Under the age of 2 years these evaluations typically include informal observational strategies, and the use of parent and professional observational checklists. As children mature, more structured standardized measures of speech and spoken or signed language come into play. These are typically administered at least once a year, and, depending upon the test battery and the child's level of communication skill, may take 2 to 10 hours. For children over the age of 3, the process of evaluation normally takes place over several sessions. Individual sessions are usually half an hour long, rarely exceed one hour and are often less. Standardized assessments of communication skills for young children are designed with motivation in mind, and, certainly, skilled clinicians exert effort to make this process enjoyable.

There is little question that children with hearing loss experience a level of structure in their preschool learning experience that exceeds that of most hearing children. A significant part of this relates to the perceived need by professionals and often by parents to engage in an assessment process that allows for the appropriate and timely targeting of communication goals. This process has been supported by legislation in the United States and other countries through the use of Individual Family Service Plans (IFSP) and Individual Program Plans (IPP), required to secure funding for Early Intervention and Special Education. IFSPs and IPPs require the setting of specific goals and the monitoring of their outcomes, which feeds directly into the assessment process. The impact of intervention activities upon normal family life and upon the emotional and social development of the child has received some attention in the early intervention literature (Shonkoff, Hauser-Cram, Krauss & Upshur, 1992) because these issues are common across disabilities in young children. Very little of this literature focuses on the social-emotional impact of evaluation, and it is from the social-emotional arena that ethical issues often arise.

There is ongoing debate about the ethical implications of using instruments standardized on hearing children to describe the communication status of children with hearing loss. Ethical questions in this arena are often linked to validity issues. Valid and ethical choices of assessment instrument depend upon the purpose for which the assessment is to be used (Messick, 1989). If a child is in an integrated setting, and the norms to which the child's parents aspire are hearing norms, then use of hearing normed instruments, always with a written statement acknowledging the lack of norms for hearing impairment, may be appropriate. If parents desire information about how their child compares with other children with hearing loss, then hearing-impaired normed instruments are appropriate. Ethical and valid choices regarding assessment processes and instruments become paramount when the results of the assessments have funding or placement decisions.

Our purpose in this chapter is not to attempt to provide solutions to the many possible ethical dilemmas that arise from the assessment process. Indeed, the entire space of this book would be inadequate for that purpose. Because of the political, and many would argue cultural, issues surrounding assessment for individuals with hearing loss, what might be identified as an ethical conflict by one person or group may not be considered as a conflict by others. Therefore, we believe that it will be most beneficial to focus our discussion on current ethical approaches as they might be applied to finding the best resolution for the wide array of ethical issues concerning assessment that might be identified by concerned stakeholders in the process.

APPROACHES TO ETHICAL DECISION MAKING

In this chapter we will illustrate the difficulties in reaching satisfactory solutions to the ethical issues in assessment faced by clinicians based on principlism, which is currently the most applied approach in bioethics. We will also sensitize our readers to other ethical approaches that may be useful in considering the ethical dilemmas that clinicians face. These include feminism and narrative approaches. We recognize, as clinicians ourselves, that at the end of the day we are called upon to make decisions with or on behalf of our clients and their families. Our intent here, however, is to offer our readers an opportunity to consider a range of possible approaches to ethical decision-making and to gain an awareness of the process. What follows then, is an invitation to view the epistemology of bioethics.

Principlism

Commonly, the ethical issues in assessment in sensory technologies are framed in the language of benefits and harms, autonomy, fair distribution, and in the case of children, best interests. Readers are most likely familiar with the principle-centered approach that undergrids this discourse. Proponents of this approach offer four ethical principles derived from various fundamental ethical theories. Beauchamp and Childress, the main proponents of this approach, have abandoned the project of developing a grand theory in favor of a mid-level approach more closely attuned to the aim of bioethics to resolve real concerns in day-to-day practice (Beauchamp & Childress, 1994; Also see Arras, 1994). They have distilled what they believe are the four ethical principles that are fundamental to health care practice (and likely education as well). These four principles are respect for autonomy, beneficence, nonmaleficence, and justice.

Autonomy, or more specifically in Beauchamp and Childress' approach, respect for autonomy, is derived from deontological theory that accords moral significance to the individual. The notion of autonomy is based on the ideals of self-determination, authenticity, and free action. The respect accorded the individual as an autonomous agent is the foundation for the principle of respect for autonomy. This respect focuses on recognizing the individual's abilities and perspectives on life (i.e., values, views, and choices). Respect for autonomy is demonstrated when the clinician recognizes the client's inherent worth irrespective of the client's life circumstances. The clinician will seek to act in a manner that facilitates the client's autonomous expression.

The principle of respect for autonomy achieved prominence in modern bioethics within the changing context of the physician-patient relationship. Traditionally, the principle of beneficence dominated ethical action in health care. However, increases in medical and scientific knowledge, technological advances, the civil rights movement, and consumer advocacy have effectively facilitated a recognition of the autonomy principle as a means of empowering the patient in this relationship. This emphasis on the principle of respect for autonomy is demonstrated in collaborative models of treatment, family-centered approaches, and the emergence of partnership models for clients, their families, and service providers. The ethical principle of respect for autonomy forms the basis for the legal doctrine of informed consent.

Limits to the principle of respect for autonomy are imposed when, in certain circumstances, it is morally justifiable to restrict autonomy in matters of public safety or distribution of scarce resources. These restrictions rest on the evocation of competing principles such as beneficence and justice (Beauchamp & Childress, 1989).

Beneficence is the ethical principle that guides us to do good. This principle is the hallmark of health care practice. Health care professionals are called upon to act in ways that positively benefit their clients. Historically, beneficence was the sole ethical imperative for medical practitioners. Changes in society and in health care described previously precipitated a turn from a reliance on an interpretation of beneficence that permitted physicians to act without consultation with the patient: Paternalism.

Nonmaleficence is the principle that obliges us to "do no harm." Some philosophers do not draw a distinction between nonmaleficence and beneficence. Rather, they claim a continuum exists. Frankena (1973), for example, argues that nonmaleficence is but one of four elements of beneficence that includes not inflicting harm, preventing harm, removing harm, and promoting good. Beauchamp and Childress (1994), in contrast, state that not inflicting harm is the essence of nonmaleficence since it involves the prevention of a negative act, whereas the remaining three elements of Frankena's schema involve positive acts that can be identified as beneficent.

Defining harm is, of course, problematic for ethicists as well as clinicians. Beauchamp and Childress (1989) offer the following definition: "[] the thwarting, defeating, or setting back of the interests of one party by the invasive actions of another party" (p. 124). As clinicians or educators in the field of communication disorders, we need to examine the concept of harm. While few situations in our practice provide the opportunity to inflict *physical* harm, the impact of our actions on the right to self-determination of the client's quality of life is open to interpretation and debate.

Justice refers to the fair distribution of benefits and burdens in a society. Theories of justice attempt to account for what the distribution ought to be. In bioethics, the debate over what constitutes a fair distribution is contentious.

The principles are not rank ordered in terms of a priority listing. Beauchamp and Childress (1994) argue that only when confronted with an ethical problem can we decide which principle deserves our attention. Beauchamp (1994) offers that the principles are intended merely as starting points from which we then move on to specification and balancing. In this sense, Beauchamp is addressing one of the criticisms of this approach which charges that the principles are vague or content thin. He defends his approach by noting that specification will involve a dialectic of considered judgments and considered principles that is drawn from John Rawls's reflective equilibrium (Rawls, 1971).

Beauchamp (1994) argues that principles structure ethical judgments to keep them from drifting toward arbitrariness. Principles are then action guides. They are "general norms of conduct that describe obligations, permissible actions, and ideals of action" (p. 955). At the same time, Beauchamp states that what is needed in a situation of conflict is "an exercise of judgment" (p. 957). Specification will involve a discussion process that serves to unpack our biases and assumptions and bring in details of the case at hand to render "contextually relevant norms" (p. 960).

Principlism has come under criticism in the field of bioethics primarily for its incompleteness and indeterminacy. In what follows, we will discuss highlights from the critiques of this dominant approach in bioethics that focus on principlism's assumption of a priori knowledge, its vagueness in defining the four principles, and its inability to effectively deal with broader issues at play in health care and educational encounters. Our case to consider is illustrative of some of the strengths and weaknesses commonly associated with the approach.

When we take a principle-centered approach to our case, we are at first confronted with the dilemma, from the clinician's perspective, of wanting to respect the mother's choice not to use invasive measures to treat her daughter's hearing impairment while at the same time wanting to do good, in this case, defined clinically as pursuing a program of aural rehabilitation that may include cochlear implantation. On first gloss, this interpretation, common enough in the professional literature on ethics (Rothman, 1991) places the dilemma in terms of deciding between two competing principles, respect for autonomy and beneficence. We will argue that while, at first, it appears that these two principles compete, the difficulty in Sara's case turns on issues of interpretation of the ethical imperative to respect individual choice.

Informed consent is the legal requirement that expresses the ethical principle of respect for autonomy. When dealing with infants and young children in the health care setting in particular, we look to their parents to make decisions on the children's behalf. Generally, we think of parents as the appropriate decision makers for their children. Social order depends to a large extent on this assumption. In the law, parents are recognized as decision makers for their child and have a responsibility to act to protect their child's interests. Only when the child's life is threatened in some fundamental way, do we, in a democratic society, step in and take control. In order to override the right of the parents to decide on behalf of their children, we must be able to demonstrate that either the parents are not competent decision makers or that their objections are unjustifiable.

Given the general recognition of the respect for autonomy principle by clinicians as evidenced by their commitment to the tenets of family-focused intervention, we must wonder why the clinician in Sara's case is uncomfortable with following through. Her discomfort may have two interpretations. First, the clinician may truly be committed to her program, including cochlear implantation, because she sees it as a biomedical good. In this case, she will be tempted to make repeated efforts to convince the parent to acquiesce. In this sense, she is seeking to override the principle of respect for autonomy on the grounds that the benefit afforded to the child exceeds any other considerations. There are two considerations to this interpretation.

The First Interpretation

Although it is true that the results of interventions can be demonstrated to be positive, the determination of benefit in an individual case requires a more nuanced and concerted effort. Results are not necessarily the same as benefits because the determination of benefits involves an assessment not only of the technical data but also consideration of the specific client's life context (Muirhead, James & Griener, 1995). On this point, the clinician will need more information from the family about their values, their priorities, and the resources available to them both from the medical and home communities. Still, an argument over benefits will unlikely result in sufficient weight being given to tip the balance in favor of the clinician's interpretation of benefit.

A second problem with the clinician's biomedical good position exposes a limitation in principlism itself. A moral language is required in order to begin discussing ethical issues. One of the early tasks is to define or at least reach some agreement on definitional issues. For example, in the area of tube feeding, speech-language pathologists and other health care professionals have struggled about whether tube feeding should be called a medical treatment, in which case it can be discontinued, or humane care, in which case, it cannot. Hoffmaster (1994) notes that you cannot begin to negotiate a solution without first settling this issue because the chosen definition will then guide your choice of applicable principles and norms. In deafness, we are aware that there is a debate about whether or not deafness is a disability. Lacking a shared understanding of deafness as a difference or a disability will make some ethical issues in deafness difficult if not impossible to settle. What strikes you as an ethical issue will depend largely on a priori knowledge and assumptions that form a moral starting point, a moral view, for all else that follows (Wildes, 2000).

The Second Interpretation

Even when the clinician recognizes Sara's mother's right to make decisions for Sara, the clinician may remain uncomfortable. How does respect for autonomy play out? This concern goes to the heart of another critique of principlism. Precisely what do any of the principles mean when we have to put them to use in ethical decision making?

One interpretation of respect for autonomy would have us accept Sara's mother's decisions without challenge. Assuming that Sara's mother is a rational free agent who acts without coercion or influence, once she is given the necessary information, she can be left alone to decide for Sara. These traits of rationality and detachment are assigned to the autonomous decision maker in our society. The clinician may intuitively realize that such a person has rarely, if ever, crossed the threshold of his or her clinic. In fact, the clinician will find support for this intuition in feminist critiques of principlism. Principlism does not offer guidelines for the patient or family member who is vulnerable, afraid, lacking information, and wanting to please the professionals who are providing care for her child. In fact, illness and disability can compromise your ability to act autonomously and can leave you open to exploitation (Sherwin, 1992).

Sherwin points out that without a deeper understanding of autonomy we may only be protecting the mechanism, informed consent, that operates to get patient agreement. In our case, we need to be very careful in the assessment process that we are not using informed consent as a way to "secure the compliance of docile patients" (Sherwin, 1992, p. 29).

Certainly, as health care professionals, we know that we cannot abandon our clients (see relevant Codes of Ethics for injunctions against abandonment). Instead, the clinician must navigate a course that respects parents' decisions while providing unbiased information and avoiding misuse of the authority and power he or she recognizes they have. This is the real challenge—to engage with families while at the same time recognizing that power may not be equalized and that those with power ought to use it ethically (Christie & Hoffmaster, 1986).

So far, we have only dealt with the outlined case from the clinician's perspective. Even if we only take the clinician's perspective, we can see that there are insufficient grounds to override the respect for autonomy that forms the ethical foundation of family-centered care. So, despite the clinician's misgivings about what she thinks is good for Sara, she must recognize her ethical obligation to respect Sara's mother's decision. This conclusion can be arrived at without casting a shadow over the wisdom of Sara's mother's decisions. While this is the ethically defensible stand, the clinician will not be without misgivings about the outcome for this child, her mother, and others in the family. As Griener states, "The downside of family-centered care is that it occasionally calls on professionals to achieve less than they might" (Muirhead, James, & Griener, 1995, p. 192).

Alternate Perspectives

In this next section, we will take up a version of Sara's mother's perspective to further illustrate the need for close examination of ethical principles in context. In order to do so, we will introduce the reader to two alternate perspectives in bioethics, feminist and narrative ethics.

A Feminist Perspective

The intent of respect for autonomy is to protect and clarify patients' rights to make their own decisions and to ensure that information is given. Generally, respect for autonomy allows us to resolve problems in favor of the patient when values collide or when those values cannot be known. The appeal for feminist bioethicists is in the principle's promise of protection for vulnerable populations that feminists identify as having experienced domination and oppression in the health care or other systems. Feminist analysis reveals that certain groups—for example, the poor, immigrant women, and people of color—are more likely to experience illness and disability. Feminists are attentive to the ways in which these particular groups have their "authority and credibility ... undermined" (Sherwin, 1998, p. 23).

From the feminist perspective in bioethics, Sherwin (1998) notes that the construction of rationality is such that some groups in our society will be seen as not capable owing to their perceived lack of objectivity and emotional distance. Interestingly, when people with disabilities act in the very ways traditionally articulated by the autonomy principle (i.e., objective and rational), we often react by putting them back into the role prescribed for them as sick or, in the case of disabled women, infantilized (Fine & Asch, 1988). We may also describe them as abrasive, pushy, and angry in an attempt to maintain the social hierarchy of medicine.

Sherwin (1998) counters the concern about this construction of rationality with a new conception of autonomy that is relational. Her relational account acknowledges that we are all socially situated. Our relationships, both with each other and with social institutions, affect how we develop our autonomy. Sherwin would reinterpret respect for autonomy in light of the conditions of choice, the available choices, and the opportunities that socialization allows to practice autonomy skills.

Sara's mother, in her narrative, reveals a decision-making process that reflects the relational configuration Sherwin seeks. This mother wonders about the effects of the proposed interventions on her whole family. She speaks of their vulnerability and her solitude/isolation as she strives to make a decision while separated from her family. As part of her decision-making process, she embraces her emotionality and her spirituality rather than dismissing it as subjective or irrelevant.

On the basis of historical oppressions, Sara's mother may be more reluctant than other families to assert a choice that challenges authority. She may know from previous experience that we are more likely to intervene when a family disagrees with us. Sara's mother may resist for reasons that she does not mention to the clinician. She may remember how children were removed from her community to be cared for by strangers in distant locales or how parents of these children were characterized as incompetent on the basis of their race, culture, or linguistic heritage. Sara's mother may know that the competencies that she and her family value are not similarly valued by other communities or that these competencies can only be revealed in particular contexts. She may also be aware that women and children have not fared well in health care despite their overrepresentation as health care consumers (Sherwin, 1992, 1998; also see Hillyer, 1993).

When we take seriously the feminist critique of principlism, we expose the weakness of a conception of autonomy grounded in rationality.

Narrative Approaches

As clinicians, we collect stories and we tell them. Stories, or narratives as they are referred to in the bioethics literature, have received attention for their role in ethics. Note that cases are really a particular form of narrative usually told from the medical perspective. Stories are an integral part of ethical discourse. Murray (1997) writes that our stories condition our ethical responses. The telling of stories raises important questions about what stories tell us about ethical life.

Narrative approaches to ethical issues in health care offer the opportunity to invite people traditionally on the periphery of power to offer their perspectives. Historically, the interpretation of illness and disability has been the health care professional's prerogative. In other words, as Arthur Frank (1997) comments, the people with power are often the ones giving meaning to others' experience. Postmodernism reminds us that one story cannot stand in for all. To take multiculturalism and plurality seriously, we must abandon the project of developing one grand narrative. We cannot arrive at shared moral meanings when a particular meaning dominates and renders all others invisible.

Might there be a different interpretation of the case from Sara's mother's perspective? Yes, this is undoubtedly possible. As we have seen in discussing the feminist perspective, it is possible for different people in different social positions to have different interpretations. This challenge to a unified moral perspective is inevitable in a pluralistic, multicultural society such as ours (Wildes, 2000). Indeed, clinicians working in deafness are familiar with this struggle to accommodate multiple and disparate voices.

It is doubtful that narrative approaches on their own have sufficient resources to resolve ethical issues in health care (Arras, 1997). At some level, narratives will require the resources offered by bioethical approaches such as principlism. However, it is recognized that they serve an important function in displacing the hegemonic discourse that has been damaging to certain groups in our society.

CONCLUSIONS

Our case demonstrates that the principle of respect for autonomy requires considerable thought as to what we mean. Indeed, as our essay illustrates, the four principles in this approach to bioethics are not self-evident. In fact, to think so, exposes the power structures of health care where one view, the one belonging to authority, prevails. The initial appeal of principlism is the appearance of objectivity suggested by the familiar presentation of principles as action guides. Clinicians may remark, like the medical student quoted by Arras (1994), "It's really objective ... just like science" (p. 993). In this essay, we have argued that ethical questions are not well served by surface understandings of ethical principles. Clinicians need to be willing and able to engage a broad array of ethical perspectives in order to craft ethically defensible solutions to the complex issues arising from the early assessment process.

REFERENCES

Arras, J. (1994). The role of cases in bioethics. *Indiana Law Journal, 69,* 983–1013.

Arras, J. (1997). Nice story, but so what? In H. Lindemann-Nelson (Ed.), *Stories and their limits* (pp. 65–88). New York: Routledge.

Fine, M., & Asch, A. (Eds.). (1988). *Women with disabilities: Essays in psychology, culture and politics* (Health, Society and Policy Series). Philadelphia: Temple University Press.

Beauchamp, T. L. (1994). Principles and other emerging paradigms in bioethics. *Indiana Law Journal, 69,* 955–971.

Beauchamp, T. L., & Childress, J. F. (1989). *Principles of biomedical ethics* (3rd ed.). New York: Oxford University Press.

Beauchamp, T. L., & Childress, J. F. (1994). *Principles of biomedical ethics* (4th ed.). New York: Oxford University Press.

Christie, R. J., & Hoffmaster, C. B. (1986). *Ethical issues in family medicine.* Oxford: Oxford University Press.

Frank, A. W. (1997). *The wounded storyteller: Body, illness, and ethics.* Chicago: University of Chicago Press.

Frankena, W. K. (1973). *Ethics* (2nd ed.). Englewood Cliffs, NJ: Prentice-Hall.

Gabbard, S. A., Thompson, V., & Brown, M. A. (1998, December). Considerations for newborn hearing screening, audiological assessment and intervention. *Audiology Today.*

Geers, A., & Moog, M. S. (Eds.). (1994). Effectiveness of cochlear implants and tactile aids for deaf children: The sensory aids study at Central Institute for the Deaf. *The Volta Review, 96*(5), 1–231.

Hellman, S. A., Chute, P. M., Kretchmer, R. E., Nevins, M. E., Parisier, S. C., & Thurston, L. C. (1991). The development of the Children's Implant Profile. *American Annals of the Deaf/Reference, 136*(2), 77–81.

Hillyer, B. (1993). *Feminism and disability.* Norman, OK: University of Oklahoma Press.

Hoffmaster, B. (1994). The forms and limits of medical ethics. *Social science and medicine, 39*(9), 1155–1166.

Messick, S. (1989). Validity. In R. Linn (Ed.), *Educational measurement* (3rd ed), (pp. 13–103). New York: American Council on Education and Macmillan Publishing Company.

Muirhead, E. S., James, P. L., & Griener, G. G. (1995). Clinical ethics forum: An examination of principle-centred decision-making in human communication disorders. *Journal of Speech-Language Pathology and Audiology, 19*(3), 187–196.

Murray, T. (1997). What do we mean by "narrative ethics"? In H. Lindemann-Nelson (Ed.), *Stories and their limits* (pp. 3–17). New York: Routledge.

Paulette, L. (1993). A choice for K'aila. *Humane Medicine, 9*(1), 13–17.

Rawls, J. (1971). *A theory of justice.* Cambridge: Harvard University Press.

Rothman, D. J. (1991). *Strangers at the bedside: A history of how law and bioethics transformed medical decision making.* New York: Basic Books.

Sherwin, S. (1992). *No longer patient: Feminist ethics and health care.* Philadelphia: Temple University Press.

Sherwin, S. (1998). A relational approach to autonomy in health care. In S. Sherwin, *The politics of women's health: Exploring agency and autonomy.* Philadelphia: The Feminist Health Care Ethics Research Network. Temple University Press.

Shonkoff, J. P., Hauser-Cram, P., Krauss, M., & Upshur, C. (1992). Development of infants with disabilities and their families. *Monographs of the Society for the Research in Child Development, 57*(6 Serial No. 230).

Waltzman, S. B., & Cohen, N. L. (Eds.). (2000). *Cochlear implants.* New York: Thieme.

Wildes, K. W. (2000). *Moral acquaintances: Methodology in bioethics.* Notre Dame: University of Notre Dame Press.

Yoshinaga-Itano, C. (1998). *Predictors of successful outcome for deaf and hard of hearing infants and toddlers.* Report presented at the NIDCD Advisory Board, NIH, 5–97.

Yoshinaga-Itano, C., Sedey, A., Coulter, D., & Mehl, A. (1998). The language of early and later identified children with hearing loss. *Pediatrics, 102*(5), 1161–1171.

FURTHER READINGS[5]

Farrell, P. M., & Fost, N. C. (1989). Long-term mechanical ventilation in pediatric respiratory failure: Medical and ethical considerations. *American Review of Respiratory Disease, 140,* S36–S40.

Hoffmaster, B. (1990). Morality and the social sciences. In G. Weisz (Ed.), *Social science perspectives on medical ethics* (pp. 241–260). Boston: Kluwer Academic.

Hoffmaster, B. (1992). Can ethnography save the life of medical ethics? *Social Science and Medicine, 35*(12), 1421–1431.

Jennings, B. (1990). Ethics and ethnography in neonatal intensive care. In G. Weisz (Ed.), *Social science perspectives on medical ethics* (pp. 261–272). Boston: Kluwer Academic.

Jonsen, A., Siegler, M., & Winslade, W. (1992). *Clinical ethics.* New York: McGraw-Hill.

Lindemann-Nelson, H. (1997). *Stories and their limits.* New York: Routledge.

Lindemann-Nelson, H., & Lindemann-Nelson, J. (1995). *The patient in the family.* New York: Routledge.

Morse, J. M., & Field, P. A. (1995). *Qualitative research methods for health professionals.* Thousand Oaks, CA: Sage.

Oliver, M. (1996). *Understanding disability: From theory to practice.* New York: St. Martin's Press.

Patton, M. (1990). *Qualitative evaluation and research methods* (2nd ed.). Newbury Park, CA: Sage.

Purtilo, R. B. (1988). Ethical issues in teamwork: The context of rehabilitation. *Archives of Physical Medicine and Rehabilitation, 69,* 318–322.

Sharp, H. M., & Genesen, L. B. (1996). Ethical decision-making in dysphagia management. *American Journal of Speech-Language Pathology, 5*(1), 15–22.

Strauss, A., & Corbin, J. (1998). *Basics of qualitative research: Grounded theory procedures and techniques* (2nd ed.). Thousand Oaks, CA: Sage.

Wolf, S. M. (Ed.). (1996). *Feminism and bioethics: Beyond reproduction.* New York: Oxford University Press.

APPENDIX A

Important or Main Points

- Essentially all children with hearing losses are assessed or evaluated—most would be extensively tested.

- Audiological assessment ranges from the innocuous observation of a child's behavior to sound stimuli in the environment, to procedures that require sedation for children over 6 months of age. Language assessment is also a common experience for children with hearing losses—ethical issues in this area are possibly more subtle.
- The ethical issues for discussion center around informed consent, resource allocation, and the child and parent's rights and best interests, or perhaps in extreme cases—harm minimization.
- Clinicians committed to family-centered practice frequently experience ethical conflict in their efforts to respect family priorities when those priorities run counter to the clinician's understanding of best clinical practice for the child.
- Following assessment there is a second reality for children with hearing losses and their parents: Hearing testing leads to assistive listening adaptations or technology designed to improve children's access to sound. Some may be innocuous as in the case of preferred seating. Other options like conventional hearing aids, FM systems, and cochlear implants may have significant resource allocation consequences for the family and life-altering consequences for the child in terms of communication method and cultural affiliation.
- During the preschool years many pedagogically and ethically based judgments are formulated relative to placement and language of instruction. Although these judgments are usually arrived at over a period of diagnostic treatment following assessment, they may still result in accusations from parents and professionals such as, "They've wasted two years trying to teach this child to speak." or "That signing child's auditory potential has been neglected."

Follow-up References or Suggestions

Text Based Materials

- Bowe, F. G. (1995). Ethics in early childhood special education. *Infants and Young Children, 7*(3), 28–37.
- Crouch, R. A. (1997). Letting the deaf be Deaf: Reconsidering the use of cochlear implants in prelingually deaf children. *The Hastings Center Report, 27*(4), 14–21.
- Estabrooks, W. (1998). *Cochlear implants for kids.* Washington, DC: Alexander Graham Bell Association for the Deaf.
- Garstecki, D. C. (2000). Morals, ethics, laws and clinical audiologists. *Seminars in Hearing, 21*(1), 21–31.
- Grant, C. (1996). Turning point: A short story. *The CAEDHH Journal, 22*(1), 4–8.
- Lane, H., & Grodin, M. (1997). Ethical issues in cochlear implant surgery: An exploration into disease, disability, and the best interests of the child. *Kennedy Institute of Ethics Journal, 7*(3), 231–251.
- Ling, D. (1988). *Foundations of spoken language for hearing impaired children.* Washington, DC: Alexander Graham Bell Association for the Deaf.

- Newman-Ryan, J. (2000). History of professional health care ethics. *Seminars in Hearing, 21*(1), 3–20.
- Ramsey, C. L. (2000). Ethics and culture in the deaf community response to cochlear implants. *Seminars in Hearing, 21*(1), 75–86.
- Robbins, A. M., Svirsky, M., Osberger, M. J., & Pisoni, D. B. (1998). Beyond the audiogram: The role of functional assessment. In F. Bess & J. Gravel (Eds.), *Children with hearing impairments: Contemporary trends* (Chapter 8). Nashville, TN: Bill Wilkerson Press.
- Tucker, B. P. (1998). Deaf culture, cochlear implants and elective disability. *The Hastings Center Report,* July–August.
- Zimmerman-Phillips, S., Osberger, M. J., & Robbins, A. M. (1997). *Infant-Toddler Meaningful Auditory Integration Scale (IT-MAIS).* Sylmar, CA: Advanced Bionics Corporation.

Videotapes

- Weisberg, R. (Producer). (2000). *Sound and Fury* [Videorecording]. Loganhulme, QLD: Marion Projects.

Ethical Questions for Consideration

- Given that most professionals in the field of deafness are strongly aligned with specific belief systems, are they ethically bound to identify their own biases in their assessment and counseling with families, as opposed to portraying a stance of "objectivity" that is highly unlikely to exist?
- Are the mother's interests different than the child's? Or put differently, is doing good (benefience) only directed at the child? Couldn't it also be interpreted as doing what is in the family's best interest?
- If parents do not consent to assessment procedures which, to the clinician's best knowledge, will make a significant difference to the child's well-being, are clinicians ethically bound to inform parents of the potential harm of refusal or delay?
- What is the clinician's ethical responsibility to the child when the parents choose not to act on the results of assessment information, or choose a course that the clinician believes is clearly not supported by the assessment results, (e.g., choosing to integrate a 6-year-old profoundly deaf child who has a 5-year language delay.)
- "Assessed to death" and "not another test" are frequent comments from parents and teachers of children with a hearing loss. How should we achieve the balance between the "need to know" and a "right to peace"?
- In the case of implantation—the ethical considerations are huge: informed consent, child and parental rights, professional obligations to inform families of their options, and such. What is the best approach to arrive at "in the best interests of the child" arrangement?
- Van Hasselt questioned, What are the ethical implications of proceeding with a cochlear implant when the proper conditions of support or follow-up

are knowingly absent? (Refer to Van Hasselt, A. (2000) *Cochlear implants in developing countries.* Paper at the 19th International Congress on Education of the Deaf and 7th Asia-Pacific Congress on Deafness [July 11]. Sydney, Australia.)

APPENDIX B

Steps in the Audiological Assessment Process

The assessment process:

- See Gabbard, Thompson, and Brown (1998) for a detailed description of this process.
- Tympanometry can be performed when the child is awake or asleep. It involves the insertion of a soft foam probe onto the child's ear canal, and takes less than 5 minutes when the child is cooperative. This test provides information about the mobility of the middle ear and allows the audiologist to form conclusions about the middle ear function. If middle ear function is abnormal, the other two electrophysiological (OAE & ABR) tests will be affected.
- The Otoacoustic Emission (OAE) test requires insertion of a soft foam insert headphone into the child's ear canal. The function of the outer hair cells of the cochlea are assessed by measuring the emission resulting from a presentation of a sound stimulus. If the child is quiet, this test can be done in as little as 15 minutes. If no emissions are evident, a sensorineural hearing loss may be suspected. This must be confirmed by Auditory Brainstem testing (ABR).
- ABR testing takes longer than the previous two measures—often 1 to 3 hours. Children older than 6 months are usually sedated for this test. Sedation is prescribed by a doctor, administered orally, and the child's status is monitored by medical personnel throughout the test. Several contact electrodes are attached in specific locations on the child's head by means of a gentle adhesive that is easily removed. Sound stimuli are presented through headphones to each ear, and the brainstem's electrical responses are averaged and graphed. The results are available and interpreted to the parents immediately following the test. OAE and ABR testing are typically done only once.
- Behavioral testing is sometimes used as a screen or, more often with the advent of OAE, as confirmation of ABR results. Very young children will often still, stop sucking on a bottle, or even search for a sound source. Prior to the advent of ABR testing, this was the only way audiologists had of determining hearing status for infants. It is much less reliable than ABR testing.
- If children are beginning to search for sound, Visual Reinforcement Audiometry (VRA) may be a more reliable behavioral test. Children are reinforced in their searching by brightly lit, moving toys that the audiologist activates when children search appropriately. When children learn the loca-

tion of the toys, they look in the appropriate direction when they hear a sound from either speakers or, preferably, insert headphones. Children as young as 18 months may develop enough consistency with this technique to provide fairly reliable results.

- The most reliable behavioral results are achieved through Play Audiometry. In this task, children hold an object up to their ear, and perform a task with the object (e.g., putting in a puzzle piece, dropping a marble in water) when they hear a sound. As children become more experienced in this task, it becomes easier to determine the child's actual threshold—the quietest sounds that they can hear. Some 2-year-olds are able to do this task, although they are usually unable to persist with it for more than a few minutes. Children over the age of 3 are frequently quite consistent in performing this task, and will perform it many hundreds of times over the course of their lives.
- In order to be certain that a child's amplification is optimal, an accurate audiogram based on consistent behavioral results is necessary. This requires repeated, consistent responses, in both ears, across all of the speech frequencies (250, 500, 1000, 2000, 4000 Hz at a minimum). Prior to obtaining this information, audiologists are able to make good estimates about the most appropriate amplification equipment and settings for the child, but they cannot be certain that they are optimal.

NOTES

[1] We are grateful for the technical counsel of Sue Hudson-Peters, MSc and Kathy Packford, MSc on matters pertaining to audiological assessment.

[2] Eleanor Stewart wishes to gratefully acknowledge the support her mother, Gwyneth Stewart, and of the Social Sciences and Humanities Research Council for support of her Doctoral studies.

[3] Kathryn Ritter's contribution was supported by the Capital Health Authority, Department of Communication Disorders at Glenrose Rehabilitation Hospital in Edmonton, Alberta, Canada.

[4] We are indebted to Paulette (1993) for the concept behind our case study.

[5] The items in this Bibliography were influential in the development of this chapter, but not directly referenced or cited. They are included here for the interest of the readers.

PART

II

FROM THREE TO
SIX YEARS

Part II, this second quartet of chapters, reflects ethical issues pertinent to the education of older preschool children with hearing losses and their families. Specifically the age range from 3 to 6 years is where the focus begins, although the chapters do have a wider perspective than the specified 3 or 4 years. In these chapters topics concerning educational programs access, the available "school" options, the curriculum considerations, and the training and competencies of teachers for children with hearing losses are featured. Like Part I, chapter coordination was considered, but having a stand-alone characteristic was seen as desirable because it would allow the reader with a particular interest to read selectively.

Chapter 6 by A. Weisel concerns early parental choice in educational placement for their child with a hearing loss. In development, I thought of this chapter as one where the decisions made and the efforts given to learning a language at home with parents would be held up for scrutiny when the child enters a formal program for language learning and education. I also though of it as a transition time—the child emerging from the "informal home" and entering the "formal school" with all the ethically related judgments of

placement and language of instruction. Weisel, by discussing ethics
of equality, excellence, and parental choice for children with hearing losses in Israel, broadened my thinking. The restricted world of
a deaf child and his or her parents, and *a* location and its resources
must always be viewed against the backdrop of group, government,
and even national agendas—religious and cultural backgrounds,
larger political realities and laws, and even founding national ideals.
Weisel's discussion of the Israeli context highlights these points
beautifully, and the bridge to other countries and settings and their
unique characteristics is not difficult.

W. McCracken's chapter also explores the topic of educational
placement for children with hearing impairments. The text includes
elements from the previous chapter but the context changes to the
United Kingdom, and the ethical "devil is in the detail." Although
Weisel made me broaden my perspective—McCracken made me
dust off the trinkets of educational placement. The "early considerations" of Deaf parents, initial placement, and school entry are discussed first. Subsequently, two frameworks relative to educational
placement and provision are considered: the political framework
and the legislative framework. A host of topics are covered under
these umbrellas—communication mode, inclusion, individual support, pragmatic perspective, practicalities, school settings or nature,
and support for learning. Family friendly services receive an
extended discussion. Subtopics include the practical approach, role
of Deaf adults, and self-esteem to mention half. The final topics of
outcome measurement and deaf children with disabilities pulls
together those areas often forgotten.

The eighth chapter by G. Leigh is introduced with the statement
that "curriculum development is fundamentally a process of effective and informed decision making." This process Leigh contends
involves "decision makers who place the highest priority on the
rights and dignity of the deaf or hard of hearing students that they
serve." Following a defining of curriculum, the variations of "hidden," official, and unofficial or "actual" are given an airing. The
implications for and reality of both the "hidden" and "actual" cur-

riculum used with children with hearing losses are then discussed. The final third of the chapter concerns a listing and exploration of answers to the four questions that are fundamental to the curriculum design process relative to children with hearing losses.

D. Stewart wrote the final chapter of this quartet. The focus is ethics and the preparation of teachers of the deaf. The content reflects the broad range of teachers who work with children with hearing losses, and is not limited to the preparation of early child-hood teachers. There is a discussion of the ethics of what we teach teachers and also how we can teach ethics education and the process of making ethical decisions. The main components of the chapter use a series of case studies to illustrate the ethics of what teacher preparation programs can teach. The dilemma of doing right while being conscious of the realities of hanging on to one's job or that of another is very real for many people. The complicating factors of loyalty, obligation, choice, pressure, self-confidence are raised—so many issues that must be managed in order to do what is right.

I'm left with—from exploration comes questions. I thank the authors.

6

EQUALITY, EXCELLENCE, AND PARENTAL CHOICE IN THE EDUCATION OF DEAF AND HARD OF HEARING CHILDREN IN ISRAEL:

ETHICS AND BALANCING INDIVIDUAL, GROUP, AND NATIONAL AGENDAS

AMATZIA WEISEL

AUTHOR INTRODUCTION

In 1978, Tel Aviv University established the Hearing Impairment Program at the School of Education. This program changed the direction of my career. As an undergraduate philosophy major, I worked for a few years as a research coordinator at the school of Education before I pursued graduate studies in deaf education and then joined the faculty. As a research coordinator, I was involved in several of the school's research and development projects. These projects included the evaluation of educational reform in Israel, which aimed at the integration of students from different social, economic, and ethnic backgrounds; the development of tools for vocational counseling; the study of the structure of minority group members' social identity; the use of computers in special education; and the study of educational policy in training.

As I was considering the possibility of studying and working in the area of deaf education, I wondered how relevant these projects would be to the field. It became clear that not only were they relevant but that they embodied central issues in deaf education. The analysis of the significance of these issues to deaf education continues to be my primary research interest, as can be seen in the present chapter.

TWO CASES TO CONSIDER

Galit is a 3-year-old deaf girl who attended a public center for early education of deaf and hard of hearing (D/HH) children since her deafness was diagnosed 2 years ago. Galit spent 2 days a week in the center and 4 days in kindergarten with hearing children. The public early education center emphasizes oral communication and offers speech, language, and auditory rehabilitation. Sign language is used sporadically, mainly in the form of Signed Hebrew, and then only with a few children with very poor oral communication skills. Galit's parents want her to be educated by the Auditory-Verbal (AV) approach, which is not offered by the public center. The parents demand Galit's enrollment at a local AV private institute and that the Ministry of Education cover the cost.

Dan is a 6-year-old deaf child who graduated from kindergarten last year and will enter first grade at the beginning of the coming year. For the last 3 years Dan attended an integrative kindergarten with 5 D/HH children and 24 hearing children. A regular teacher worked in this kindergarten in addition to a teacher who specialized in the education of D/HH children. The specialized teacher knew some Israeli Sign Language (ISL) and could communicate in Signed Hebrew although most of the communication with the children was in spoken language (i.e., Hebrew). All the D/HH children used personal hearing aids and the kindergarten was acoustically adjusted for their needs. For the last 3 years Dan spent 1 day a week in a special public early educational center for D/HH children where he received individual lessons in speech, language development, and auditory training, and his achievements in these areas were quite good.

As required by the Special Education Law (SEL), Dan's case was discussed by a placement committee, before he moved to first grade. The committee decided that Dan will attend a home class for D/HH students in a regular school and will be integrated into a regular class for specific lessons according to his abilities in specific subject areas. The committee based its decision on several considerations: (1) Dan has good communication skills in both Hebrew and ISL and his presence in the special class is of high value for that class and will contribute to the social structure of the class and to its academic level. (2) Dan's affiliation with the special class will contribute to his social and emotional development. (3) It is not realistic to expect that Dan's needs will be met within a regular class in a regular school because the school has neither trained educational staff nor the resources for proper amplification and acoustic arrangements.

Dan's parents, both well-educated professionals, objected to the committee's decision and requested that Dan attend a regular class within a regular school and that the class will be acoustically adjusted. They requested that auditory and communication training be provided in a rehabilitation center that they choose and not necessarily within a public school. The parents argued that since Dan is able to cope with the regular class requirements he should not be forced to stay in the special class for D/HH students. The parents said that in the future they will consider encouraging Dan to join social and extracurricular activities with D/HH children, if necessary.

Should the demands of Galit's and Dan's parents be accepted?

INTRODUCTION

In 1999 several volunteer organizations of parents of D/HH children and professionals in the field of deaf education initiated a change in the 1988 Israeli Special Education Law (SEL). Similar to the American PL 94–142, the Israeli SEL requires the preference of regular educational settings over special ones when the educational placement of students with special needs is considered. In addition, the law gives the parents the right to participate in the process of decision making about their child's educational placement. The suggested changes in the Israeli SEL aimed to further increase the rights of the parents and their influence on the education of their children and to introduce private organizations and agencies into the system. Thus, the suggested changes of the SEL are related to several central issues that are often discussed in the sociological-educational literature. These issues include: centralization and decentralization of educational systems; duties and obligations of public educational systems; public and social interests versus individuals' rights; the relationships between public and private educational institutions and services and the degrees of parental choice with regards to educational placement, curriculum, and special education services. In the following chapter, the suggested changes of the Israeli SEL will be discussed with reference to the previously mentioned issues while examining their relevancy to the education of D/HH students. Because this discussion will be conducted in the context of the Israeli educational system, some basic information about this system will be presented first.

GENERAL INFORMATION ABOUT THE ISRAELI EDUCATIONAL SYSTEM

The Israeli population of 6.3 million people consists of the Jewish Majority (81%) and the Arab minority (19%). Almost all the educational system is run by the government and funded by public money. The educational system is divided according to the four main sectors of the Israeli population: the General Secular Jewish sector (including a small rural sector), the General Religious Jewish sector, an Ultra Orthodox Religious Jewish sector, and the Arab sector, which includes a small Bedouin community.

General Secular Jewish Sector

About 40% of the Israeli students belong to this sector. The educational system of this sector is more like the education systems in western democratic countries than the other sectors. Democratic and liberal values are relatively more pronounced in this sector. The curriculum includes regular subjects such as literature, science, mathematics, art, and history as well as Israeli and Jewish culture and heritage.

Deaf education in this sector is influenced to some extent from the various social perceptions of deafness but a medical perception is more common. Thus, oral education exists alongside Total Communication (TC). A few children are educated in the AV approach. In this sector there are special and integrative programs for D/HH students at the preschool, elementary, and secondary levels, including academic and vocational tracks. At the elementary level, about 20% of the D/HH students study in special schools, another 30% attended special classes in regular schools, and about 50% are mainstreamed. At the high school level there are special classes for D/HH students within vocational high schools. In addition there are few programs within comprehensive schools that include special classes and part-time or full-time mainstreaming, with both academic and vocational tracks. In the three larger cities in Israel there are centers that offer informal educational activities for D/HH children. D/HH adults who belong to this sector and graduated from its educational system vary considerably in their socioeconomic status, mainly according to their educational achievements (Sela & Weisel, 1992). In sum, although the available educational services in this sector do not meet all the demands, especially with regard to vocational training and informal education and particularly outside the main cities, the situation is much better than in the other sectors.

General Religious Jewish Sector

The population of this sector includes religious people, relatively conservative but modern and democratic. About 25% of the Israeli students belong to this sector. The curriculum of the educational system of this sector is shaped and supervised by the religious department in the Ministry of Education and it includes both regular subjects and a special emphasis on Jewish religious studies.

The dominant perception of deafness in the sector is the medical one without a systematic use of sign language. Children in the preschool level are educated in regular kindergartens with hearing children. There are few if any special programs for D/HH students at the high school level or any vocational programs that are part of this sector. Some of the students, in various levels of education, participate in the programs of the secular sector. In general, those D/HH students who have good communication skills in spoken language and succeed in mainstream settings enjoy reasonable status and care both as students and as adults. Those, however, who do not reach this level of achievement do not have educational services that are adjusted to their needs. As adults the hearing impaired in this sector, and especially the deaf ones, have a low and marginal social status.

Ultra-Orthodox Religious Jewish Sector

This Jewish sector, which includes about 12% of the Israeli student population, is similar in many characteristics to the State/Public Religious sector but it is more extreme in its religious lifestyle and it strongly resists any external influences. One result of this resistance is that children are never sent to study outside of the educational system of this sector. It should be noted that in both religious sectors, girls and boys study separately, a fact that causes further division within the population of D/HH students. In the preschool level there are two centers, both use an oral-only approach. Except for a few special classes, there are no special services for D/HH children at the elementary or the secondary level and no vocational training programs. The strong emphasis within this sector on religious studies, which are often the basis for social mobility, puts most of the D/HH students in a severe disadvantaged situation, since these studies require very good literacy skills. The result is that most of the students, especially the deaf ones and especially women, have, as adults, only a very marginal social status.

Arab Sector

About 19% of the Israeli population are Arabs but because of the relatively high birth rate in this sector, Arab students comprise about 23% of the total student population in Israel. The rate of D/HH children in this sector is higher than in the general population mainly because of consanguineous marriages. In this sector there is only one center for preschool education of D/HH children and some children receive services at the centers of the State/Public Secular sector. The low number of special classes at the elementary and the secondary level fails to meet the needs of the many children who are staying in regular classes without adequate services and accommodations. As adults, the D/HH and especially women, have very low social and economic status. The lack of Arab professionals—teachers, audiologists, speech pathologists, counselors, and psychologists—makes it difficult to establish adequate educational and rehabilitation services.

Follow-on Considerations

The government, by the Ministry of Education, funds most of the educational services and supervises their operation. Each educational sector, however, has a significant level of autonomy with regard to curriculum, student evaluation, staff development, and general educational policy. Naturally, there are many conflicts between the central Ministry of Education and some of the educational sectors about the degree of autonomy of each sector, the extent of the central supervision, and the involvement of the ministry in curricular issues. These conflicts are often the subject of severe political debates within the Israeli Parliament because each sector is associated with specific political orientation and ideology.

With regard to parental choice it should be noted that parents are free to select the educational sector in which their child will learn. Usually they base their choice on their social affiliation to a specific sector although there is a growing number of exceptions to this rule. In other words, there is some tendency of the different educational sectors to compete with each other for students. This competition involves educational, ideological, and political issues as well as financial ones. The existence of the different sectors reflects the acknowledgment of the founders of the state of Israel, more than 50 years ago, of the cultural diversity of the population. Therefore, within the Israeli public education system, parents have a high degree of influence on their children's education by choosing the educational sector. Within the selected sector, however, their choices are sometimes quite limited. This is especially pronounced in the relatively small sectors (e.g., the Arab sector and the Ultra Orthodox sector). In spite of the fact that the education system is government funded, there are very large differences among the sectors. Since the sectors vary with regard to the dominant social values, style of life, social and family structure, and socioeconomic status, it is difficult and often impossible to establish the same educational standards and procedures in all the sectors. The differences exist both with regard to the general student population and to the deaf student population. It should be noted that the differences among the sectors with regard to the education of D/HH children exist in despite the fact that the total number of D/HH children in Israel is quite small. It is estimated that 150 D/HH children are identified each year (Sela & Weisel, 1992). The variations in the educational services they receive depend, to a large extent, on the sector each child belongs to as well as on the specific geographical area in which she or he lives. The small but very diverse number of D/HH children makes it difficult to establish educational policy and to pass laws that are relevant and adequate to all the students.

THE ISRAELI EDUCATIONAL REFORM AND
THE SPECIAL EDUCATIONAL LAW (SEL)

The discussion about an increase in the influence of parents of D/HH children on the education of their children is carried out within a certain social and political climate. This climate is reflected in the education policy of regular and special education. Two main factors that affected the educational policy in Israel are the educational reform of the 1960s and the SEL of 1988. These two factors will be presented while considering the principles on which they are based and their approach to the issue of parental choice.

The Educational Reform

The reform of the Israeli education system at the end of 1960s and during the 1970s, like similar reforms in other western countries, was introduced to increase equality, to increase the integration between different social classes and ethnic groups and to close or reduce the gaps among them. As part of the educational reform in Israel comprehensive schools were established and students were bussed, usually from low SES neighborhoods to schools with students from higher SES background, in order to control the class compositions. The guiding principle was that in order to achieve the national goal of social integration and equality it is legitimate to limit the freedom of choice of parents and children, especially of those of upper SES.

During the 1980s, when Republicans Reagan and Bush were the U.S. presidents, the conservative Thatcher was the Prime Minister in the UK, and right-wing governments headed by Begin and then Shamir were in Israel, the central value was changed from equality to excellence. The emphasis on excellence meant that more resources were directed toward the high achieving students. Those who advocate excellence are more concerned about the average achievement in a given society whereas those who advocate equality are concerned about the distribution of achievements among various social groups. Legally, the educational policy was guided by the value of equality, as it expressed itself in the educational reform, but growing public support was given to the value of excellence. Parents from relatively high SES more easily identified with the value of excellence because their children could benefit most if this value become a dominant one. Some of these parents challenged the legal status of the educational policy, which is based on the value of equality and limits their freedom of choice. Several cases in which parents did not agree with the educational placement decisions of the educational authorities were brought to the Israeli Supreme Court.

The Rulings of the Supreme Court

Gal (1995) reviewed 13 cases, in which the issue of parental choice was evaluated in contrast to the educational policy. In general the court accepted the approach of the educational authorities although there were some differences in the ways the decisions were justified. In its 1971 decision (*Kramer v. The Municipality of Jerusalem,* in Gal, 1995) the court made it clear that the educational policy is a central means for increasing social integration and for the success of this policy it is justifiable to force the citizens to give up part of their freedom of choice. The court added that eventually the citizens will gain more than they lose because they will live in a better and more just society. In a ruling from 1977 (*Ramat Raziel Committee v. Mount Yehuda Regional Public School,* in Gal, 1997) the judge emphasized that parents have the right to choose a specific sector within their region but that they cannot select a specific school within the sector. In other words, the court ruled that within each sector the goals of the educational reform must be kept even if this means that children of higher SES background will not be able to maximize their academic achievements. In another ruling the court said clearly:

> [. . .] the plaintiffs' children will study in a school that is academically not as good as the school they expected them to join. The basis for this result has to do with the implementation of the educational policy of integration ... we understand the plaintiff's question "why do we and our children have to pay the price of this policy?" However, the answer is that someone has to carry the burden ... and, in fact, this should not be viewed as a burden only but as a right because they are fulfilling a top priority national mission. *(Hayoon v. The Mayor of Hertzelia,* 1980, in Gal, 1995, p. 208)

In a recent decision the Supreme Court rejected an appeal by 48 families of children in a city in the south region of Israel who wanted their children to study in a high school outside their area. The court accepted the mayor's argument that it is not right that high achieving students will be educated outside of the city just because their parents can pay 1200 Israeli Shekels (about $300) per month for the better education (Arbeli, 2000). By allowing these students to study outside the city, the mayor argued that the chances to improve the educational services within the city decreased.

In sum, the court consistently accepted the following principles: (1) The educational reform was accepted by the parliament and therefore it is legally a legitimate policy. (2) When there is a conflict between the individual's interest and the accepted educational policy, the interest of the public should be adopted. (3) The court accepted the assumption that educational placement is a "zero sum game" (Willms & Chen, 1989) and that some students are going to lose some of their educational opportunities. In spite of that the court ruled that this policy is justifiable in light of the important national goal it serves. (4) The pluralistic nature of the Israeli educational system was established some 50 years ago by having the different educational sectors. This structure gives the parents the freedom to choose a sector and this freedom should remain.

Although the court keeps its support for the educational policy, which was defined when the educational reform was introduced, many individuals and institutions objected to this policy. Only a few of them argued about their position by legal procedures. More often they found other ways to minimize what they considered to be the negative effects of the educational reform.

Reactions to the Educational Reform

A few different reactions to the educational policy of integration of students from different social and ethnic groups emerged. These reactions reflected parents' motivation to maximize their children's academic achievements, to shape the children's cultural and religious style of life and affiliation, and to promote specific social values and norms (Inbar, 1994). Parents from relatively heterogeneous cities, in which schools zones were clearly defined, moved to smaller cities and towns with more homogeneous populations of upper middle classes and high classes (Chen, 1997). This practice allowed the parents to ensure that their children will have a good educational and social environment without the need to openly argue against the educational authorities and without expressing general disagreement toward the values of equality and social solidarity and responsibility. In practice, the tendency to move to homogeneous cities is totally in contrast to the social goals of the educational reform. In fact, this tendency increases the differentiation among different social classes in the educational context as well as in the wider social context.

Another counterreaction to the educational reform was the establishment of special schools (Goldring, Hawley, Saffold, & Smrekar, 1997). In the United States these schools include magnet schools which are part of the public educational system, and charter schools which are for-profit organizations supervised by various public organizations (Nathan, 1997). In Israel special schools were established, mainly in the major cities by educators and parents, with each school specializing in a specific discipline such as sciences, art, communication, and even the values of the labor movement. Officially each school is required to take a specific proportion of students from different social classes in order to keep the principle of integration. Practically, however, it is doubtful if this proportion is achieved since the acceptance to one of these schools depends on the results of examinations and because parents are asked to pay for their children's education, which is otherwise free. The municipalities often give special support to these schools because they improve the prestige of the city and because they reduce the motivation of well-to-do parents to leave the city.

Other responses to the educational reform are the control-choice programs that operate in several cities in Israel and are similar to the one in Wisconsin (McGroarty, 1996). In this program parents are allowed to choose two schools, in first and second priority and the final decision about placement depends on the proportion of students from different social classes in each school. Control-choice can be seen as an attempt to keep the value of equality and the practice of social integration while giving the parents some freedom to influence the placement decisions. Advocates of this program claim that there is not a necessary contradiction between excellence and equality and that excellence does not necessarily need to be associated with elitism (Shapira, Haymann, & Shavit, 1995). Still, the empirical support for these claims is not consistent and therefore the academic and public debate about their validity continues (Goldring et al., 1997).

A voucher system is used in some countries (Alexander, 1998; Meyerson, 1999) but not in Israel (Yet!). Still, some of the suggestions to change the Israeli SEL with regard to D/HH children follow similar rationale to that of the voucher system. In this system, the students and the parents get a voucher that specifies the child's rights for remedial and special education as well as special rehabilitation services. The child and the parents can select the specific place where the services will be provided, either in the school where the child is studying or in other public or private institutions (McGroarty, 1996). The inclusion of private institutions introduces a mechanism of competition into the educational system. In order to receive the vouchers the schools have to convince the parents that they will receive good services. This competition is likely to improve the services in all the schools (Chubb & Moe, 1990, 1997).

The reactions to educational reform in Israel are similar to those of other countries and they reflect a change in the social and ideological climate in many western countries. This change includes privatization of the educational systems, considerations of this system as a free market enterprise, emphasis on excellence, and an increase in the parents' freedom of choice (Chubb & Moe, 1990). It can be asked who is going to benefit from these changes and whether these changes will improve the condition of children with special needs (Barton, 1995). In any case, the suggested changes in the Israeli SEL should be discussed while considering the changes in the social and ideological climate. Such a discussion will follow a short description of the SEL itself and the suggested changes.

The Special Education Law (SEL) 1988

The Israeli SEL, passed in 1988, is similar to the 1975 American law (PL 94-142). The two most significant parts of the law are the mandatory preference of regular educational placement over special education for students with special needs and the status of the parents in the decision-making process. Parents can participate in the meetings of the placement committee, review the documents the committee uses, have professionals as their representatives, appeal to a higher committee in cases where they disagree with the placement committee's decision, and take the case to the court. Since the parents have a strong role in the process, in most cases their position is accepted. Because the Ministry of Education usually avoids confrontations in the court, persistent parents can almost always have their way.

The educational and rehabilitation services that each group of special-needs children is entitled to are listed in the law. The availability of the services, however, often depends on the allocation of the right budget by the Ministry of Finance and by the regional authorities. The principal of the school in which a special-needs child is studying is responsible for the actual application of the services. For that purpose, the principal gets specific "teaching hours" that she or he can use either in the school or via a special regional center to provide educational and rehabilitation services. Because of the involvement of the Ministry of Finance, the local authorities (e.g., municipalities, regional councils), and the principals, in some cases there are gaps between the rights of each specific child and the actual "teaching hours" he or she gets. Furthermore, because of the need to coordinate a number of different factors, and especially between government ministries and local authorities, there are gaps between the various communities and sectors in the quantity and quality of the services the children receive.

The SEL and Parental Choice

In addition to the parents' right to participate in the decision-making process about educational placement they can be involved in curricular issues because the individual educational plan of their child must be approved by them. In fact the law gives the parents a lot of control on issues that were previously the responsibility of the educational authorities only. Long ago it was recognized that placement of children in a special education setting was biased and therefore too many children from low SES background and/or from specific ethnic groups were referred to special education (Dunn, 1968). Because of this recognition, the law, both the American and the Israeli one, requires that the placement of each individual child must be justified and that the parents will be involved. The status of the parents in the decision-making processes about educational placement and about the curriculum gives them the responsibility for quality control. And, the more the educational system is moving toward a "free market" style of operation, the more pronounced these parents' responsibilities and control become since they are the "customers." The risk in this trend is that the educational system will subordinate educational considerations to economic ones. Schmid (1986) argued that because of this risk the government and the Ministry of Education should keep the role of quality control in order to protect the "customers" (i.e., the children and the parents), and to ensure appropriate educational standards.

Considering the rights of parents of children with special needs to be involved with and to influence the education of their children it seems that as a consequence of the SEL these parents have relatively more influence on the education of their children than parents of students in regular education. Decisions about educational placement of regular students are often limited because of public considerations, whereas those regarding students with special needs are made on individual basis only. Still, it should be noted that there are limits to the choices students with special needs have as well. First, the number of different educational programs available for these students is a priori limited because of the small number of students in the various categories of special needs and in each geographical area. Second, although the court ruled that the regional council and its educational authorities must make the necessary accommodations in order to include students with special needs (*Botzer v. The Regional Council of Makabim-Reut,* 1993 in Gal, 1995), these accommodations were required only from the local school where the student belongs. It is unlikely that the court would make similar ruling with regard to any other school the student or his parents choose. It is unlikely that any student, with any special need, in any sector and geographical area will have the necessary services and facilities in any school he or she prefers. Practically and financially, such a situation is unrealistic. In the United States, for example, the Supreme Court rejected a request of a deaf student for an educational sign language interpreter both because of educational and practical reasons (*The Hendrick Hudson Central School District v. Rowley,* in Tucker, 1983; Underwood & Mead, 1995). In spite of these limitations parents of special-needs students have the right to be involved in the education of their children to a significant degree. The suggested changes in the SEL with regard to D/HH children are aimed at further increasing the rights and the freedom of choice of the parents.

SUGGESTED CHANGES OF THE SEL

The Reasons for the Changes

As mentioned in the Introduction of this chapter, in 1999 a group of parents of D/HH children, together with several Jewish and Arab volunteer organizations, including the Auditory-Verbal organization, initiated a change to the SEL. The initiators mentioned several reasons for the change:

1. In spite of the fact that the Israeli educational system is a centeralistic system and is funded by the government, there are big differences between the educational services in different geographical areas and in different sectors.

2. Different educational approaches are used in the various preschool education centers for D/HH children. For various historical reasons, and possibly because of the characteristics of the population in each region, there are centers in which sign language is used, usually in the context of TC, while other centers use the oral approach. The AV approach is not used systematically in any of the big centers— rather only by the AV volunteer organization and thus it is not funded appropriately.

3. Although there are official standards for the number of "teaching hours" each child is entitled to, these standards are not detailed enough and they do not meet the needs.

4. Although there are official standards for the number of "teaching hours" and types of educational and rehabilitation services, there are big differences among the various educational institutions in the services they actually deliver. These differences are caused by lack of professionals in specific geographical areas and sectors, and difficulties in the required coordination among various agencies.

5. The small number of D/HH in specific areas and sectors makes it even more difficult to ensure that each child will receive the services to which he or she is entitled. This is the case with regard to formal as well as to informal education.

6. Partial services are provided by organizations that were originally volunteer organizations founded by parents and professionals. These organizations are now supported by the government in addition to the funds they raise themselves. Because of the volunteer nature of these organization they are not obliged—officially, legally, and practically—to offer specific services and to offer them equally to all the D/HH children in the country.

7. In the present situation it is not possible to force the authorities to offer adequate specific educational and rehabilitation services, and the actual operation of the system is limited by financial and administrative considerations.

The Main Suggested Changes in the SEL with Regard to D/HH Children

Because of the limitations of the present situation the following suggestions were made:

1. Every child, with 25 dB hearing loss and above, is entitled to educational and rehabilitation services listed in the law in either Hebrew or Arabic (the two official languages in Israel) according to his/her parents' preference.

2. A "services basket" will be defined for each individual child according to his/her condition (e.g., severity of the condition, presence of additional handicapping conditions) and assessment of educational and rehabilitation needs. The services will include auditory rehabilitation, speech training, interpretation and note-taking services, individual educational plans, psychological and social work services, parents counseling, and the like. The individual basis for the definition of this services basket will ensure equal and universal rights. The definition of the services in the basket will be reviewed periodically and the law will be adapted accordingly. By following this procedure the separation of those who define the rights from those who have to offer the services will be established.

3. The child will be able to receive the services either in his/her school or in a public or a private educational and rehabilitation center, according to the parents' choice. The parents can also divide the services between different agencies/institutions.

4. The minister of education will define the specific rules and requirements for the educational and rehabilitation centers and will be responsible for establishing new centers wherever they are necessary.

5. The ministry of education is responsible for training professionals—teachers for D/HH children, speech pathologists, audiologists, sign language interpreters—as necessary.

The suggestions include many other details, but the main points, which are relevant to the following discussion, are the increase in the freedom of the parents to choose the educational and rehabilitation center by a voucher system and the introduction of private centers as part of the educational system. These changes are not in direct conflict with the SEL and its spirit. As mentioned earlier, the SEL already gives parents of special-needs students a relatively high degree of freedom in their involvement in the education of their children. It seems then, that the inclusion of private institutions and organizations is the main new change. The suggested changes are in line with the more general tendency to privatize various economic and social institutions, including the educational system (Chubb & Moe, 1990). It is therefore possible to evaluate this trend with regard to the education of deaf students. It can be asked whether deaf students are going to benefit from the privatization of the educational services. It can be also asked who among the deaf students will benefit most from the suggested changes.

The material presented thus far provides the necessary background about the Israeli educational system, about the educational reform of this system, and about the Israeli SEL. The suggestions to change the SEL and to increase parental choice were also presented and the broader context of privatization of the educational system was noted. Some of the assumptions and claims of those who suggested changes to the SEL and supported privatization will be presented, discussed, and challenged in the following section. In listing these assumptions and claims we used the reasons for the suggested changes and their goals that were presented earlier, as well as the arguments for and against the increase in parental choice summarized by Goldring et al. (1997).

THE FUNCTIONS OF EDUCATION AND THE FREEDOM OF CHOICE

Choice advocates claim that since parents have the responsibility to ensure that their children will be educated, it is their right to have the individual freedom to effect the education of their children. This freedom is especially relevant in the area of deaf education. Everyone familiar with the field of deaf education is aware of the old controversies about different methods of communication. It is reasonable to assume that these controversies are not going to end and that we are not going to have a clear consensus in the foreseeable future. This is perhaps because there is more than one way to perceive deafness and that the various methods reflect different philosophical and ideological perceptions. Particularly when there is no professional and/or philosophical consensus it is the duty and the right of the individual parents to make the decisions.

The discussion about parental choice involves two different approaches to the function of education. One approach sees education as a service that the state provides to its citizens. The other approach sees education as a means the state is using in order to shape the future society (Gal, 1995). The first approach perceives the students, including those with special needs and hearing impairments, on an individual basis. The second approach emphasizes the social aspects of educating groups of students. Choice advocates and those who suggested changes to the SEL in Israel, emphasize the first approach, minimize the importance of the second one, and argue that individualistic perceptions and increase in choice do not necessarily contradict the social function of education. This seems to be a matter of priority—either social goals are emphasized or individuals' rights are. It is clear that freedom of choice, by itself, is considered very differently in the two approaches. Choice advocates' argument is in clear contrast to the ideas of the educational reform and to the rulings of the Supreme Court, which clearly prefer the social function of education. In line with the preference of the social function of education, the freedom of choice of regular students is often limited.

The educational reform was based on collective values of equality and social solidarity. According to the principles of the educational reform and the court rulings, students and their parents must contribute their share to fulfill national and social missions. Within the framework of the SEL, however, students with special needs are not perceived as those who should have to shoulder their share as well. Yet, they are the ones who, because of their special needs, will benefit from the social solidarity expressed by the regular students. Is it legitimate to limit the freedom of choice of D/HH students in order to shape the future of the group of D/HH students and of the Deaf community? Is it justified to limit the freedom of choice of some D/HH students in order to establish some level of solidarity within the population of D/HH people? If education is considered as a service for the students, and in line with the SEL, the answer is no. However, if education is considered as a social means, the answer is yes.

PERCEPTIONS OF DEAFNESS

The two approaches to the function of education are related to the two central perceptions of deafness and to the communication methods associated with them. Although there is no intention to discuss the various communication methods within this chapter, the different perceptions of deafness are relevant to the present topic. The main distinction that should be noted is between the medical/audiological perception of deafness and the social one. Within the first perception, deafness is perceived as a characteristic of the individual child, a condition that involves mainly the hearing system. Within the social perception of deafness, the hearing impairment is just the basis for both social affiliation and identity and for various social attitudes toward D/HH people. The relevancy of these perceptions to educational policy was widely discussed in the literature (e.g., Bunch, 1994; Stinson & Lang, 1994) since these perceptions affect the attitudes toward the mainstreaming of D/HH students. The medical/audiological perception encourages the maximum level of integration of D/HH students with hearing students and discourages the association with other D/HH children. The social perception is geared more toward the establishment of special educational settings—special schools or special classes for D/HH students. The association between specific perception of deafness and specific approach to the function of education makes the issue a complicated one. Certainly, it is clear that parents can have their own perception of deafness. If, for example, they hold a medical/audiological perception of deafness, then it is likely that education will be perceived only as a service to the individual and no considerations would be given to D/HH students as a group. This is in clear contrast with the perception of education as a social means. It is not surprising that most of the Israeli parents who suggested changes in the SEL are educating their children in the AV approach. Thus, it seems that the opposition to parents' right to educate their children according to the medical/audiological perception of deafness may be based not on the evaluation of this perception as such but on its lack of consideration to the broader social context.

ACADEMIC ACHIEVEMENT VERSUS SOCIAL AND EMOTIONAL DEVELOPMENT

Reservations about the individualistic perception of deafness, and the consequent educational policy (i.e., mainstreaming) can be based on the influence it has on the group of D/HH students and on the future Deaf community, as was mentioned previously. In addition, it can be argued that this educational policy does not adequately ensure the social and the psychological development of the students.

Research indicated that integrative educational settings improve the academic achievement of D/HH student (Bunch, 1994; Foster, 1989; Paul & Quigley, 1990) but put a difficult social burden on these students who are often isolated and lonely (Antia, 1998). Research also indicated that the association of D/HH students with other students with hearing impairments and the use of sign language enhance emotional and social development and are related to better self-image (Bat-Chava, 1993; Stinson & Lang, 1994; Weisel, 1991, 1998). If both of these two general conclusions are valid, this means that any decision about educational placement involves potential benefits and potential risks. Parents tend to base their decision more on the potential academic advantages and therefore tend to prefer integrative placements. Some professionals, however (including the author of this chapter), who see the potential emotional and social risks can argue that it is the responsibility of the educational system to make sure that careful consideration is given to these aspects of development. One can further question if the public, by the Ministry of Education, can approve and support educational procedures that might risk the proper emotional and social development of the students. In spite of this emphasis on the social-emotional aspects of development it is doubtful if the freedom of choice of the parents should be limited on the basis of this issue alone. This is because it is quite difficult to weigh and compare the risks and the benefits that are involved—especially when the risks and benefits of a specific individual child are concerned. The answer to the hypothetical question "What would you like your child to have, higher academic achievements or better self-image?" depends on the parents' values and therefore parents should be entitled to take the risks that are involved in either decision. Still, because each decision involves potential risks, the awareness of the risks are of utmost importance. Who is responsible for informing the parents about various risks is an open question that is going to be a more central one if or when the privatization of educational services continues.

EXCELLENCE VERSUS EQUALITY

Excellence and equity are conflicting values that have competed in their influence on education policy for many years. Equity was the ideological basis for the Israeli educational reform as well as for similar reforms in other countries during the 1960s and the 1970s (e.g., Sweden, the United States, and the United Kingdom). These reforms meant integration of students of higher SES with those of a lower SES. In the 1980s, during the Reagan-Thatcher years and right-wing governments in Israel, however, educational reforms assumed a different direction: Their main theme became "excellence." Advocates of excellence are mainly concerned with the average achievement level of any given population of students. Those who emphasize equity are more concerned about the distribution of achievement levels within the population, especially with regard to various social groups (e.g., groups with low and high SES, ethnic, or racial groups).

There is a clear contrast between excellence and equity, because resources for educational investment are limited, making it impossible to invest both in *all* individuals and in the *best* schools simultaneously, and because it is likely that educational investment is a zero-sum game (Willms & Chen, 1989). The conflict between excellence and equity is basically "rooted in different social philosophies" (Bacharach, 1990, p. 418). These philosophies are used in very interesting but inconsistent ways by parents of D/HH who advocate choice.

Parents' motivation to place their D/HH children in as regular an educational setting as possible is based mainly on the value of excellence. Their main concern is that their children maximize their educational potentials. However, the student's right to study in regular educational settings is based on the value of equity. Hearing students and their parents are requested to have D/HH students in the regular classes despite the fact that such integration can negatively affect the hearing students' achievements. This is done according to the SEL and in the name of equity. In fact, it is the value of equity that makes the integration of D/HH into regular classes possible. It seems then that parents are "switching" philosophies and use equity, and the social solidarity associated with it, as well as excellence and the individualistic perception of deafness, in order to maximize their children's opportunities.

The legitimacy and the morality of the fact that some parents take advantage of the social value of equity in order to promote a competing value, excellence, can be questioned, but in any case it has some important consequences with regard to the education system of D/HH students. When integration of D/HH students is discussed, it is often assumed that the issue is about the integration of D/HH students into the hearing educational environment (Antia, 1998). It is possible, however, to consider integration *within* the D/HH population as well. Since D/HH students are a heterogeneous group that includes students from different socioeconomic backgrounds, different ability levels, and different communication skills, we can and should think about integration within this group in terms similar to those used when considering integration within the population of hearing students. Using these terms, it may be concluded that segregating the more talented D/HH students from other D/HH students by integrating them into hearing educational settings can have a negative academic impact on the D/HH students who remain in special education. This is addition to its negative impact on the social composition of the D/HH students as a whole.

Parents of D/HH children who advocate choice and follow an individualistic perception of deafness, pursuing excellence and segregation (from other D/HH students) as well as equity and integration (with hearing students), can lead to the weakening of the D/HH group. Along the way they might lose highly significant supporters in the continuous struggle for equity. It is quite possible that the solidarity of the group is an important factor in promoting equity for many individuals. In the context of privatization and its emphasis on individual excellence, losing supporters in the struggle for equity is, perhaps, not in the choice advocates' best interest.

CHOICE AND MARKETING OF COMPETING
VALUES

Choice advocates argue that increased choice will lead to competition within the educational system and will break the government monopoly in running the schools (Chen, 1997; Chubb & Moe, 1990; Goldring et al., 1997). Competition will force schools and programs to improve their services, to have better teachers, and to define marketable educational goals. Schools that work in a free market environment will have to seek a better fit between their goals and the expectations of the parents, the customers. The term "marketable educational goals" can be examined in relation to the values and perceptions, that were discussed earlier and that shape parents' expectations.

Increase of choice and privatization and especially the introduction of the voucher system go hand in hand with the values of individualism and excellence because they aim at maximizing the achievements of the individual student. Legitimate as these values are, especially from the parents' perspective, in a free market environment they might weaken the social value of equity. Some sense of social solidarity is required in order to keep social values such as equity able to compete. Chen (1997) argued that:

> The contrast between choice and equity has been evident in the frequent unwillingness of decentralized educational authorities to divert appropriate educational resources to the poor, minorities, handicapped people, and other students with special needs. Only by applying to higher levels of the legislatures, the courts, and the government, have disadvantaged groups succeeded in generating equity-based laws, leading to affirmative action. (Chen, 1997, p. 45)

According to this argument, parents of D/HH should be the last ones to promote choice since it weakens the value of equity. Unless there is an efficient mechanism by which disadvantaged groups, including D/HH people, are organized in order to be able to present their demands for equity, there is a risk that increased choice can cause more harm than good.

CHOICE, VOUCHERS, AND SOCIAL EQUALITY

Supporters of privatization claim that the introduction of competition into the general educational system will have several positive results. Results include an increase in the range of educational services in order to satisfy different groups of parents, improvement of the services in order to compete successfully, and more equal use of these services (Fox, 1999; Goldring et al., 1997). It can be asked what are the results with regard to students with special needs and D/HH students?

The experience in Germany, the United Kingdom, and Austria showed that privatization and vouchers increased both the degree of choice parents of special-needs students had, and the parents' support of full inclusion (Pijil & Dyson, 1998). However, budget limitations and difficulties in accepting students with special needs became more pronounced, especially in relatively good regular schools. Increase in parental choice caused relatively poor schools to accept more students with special needs compared with good schools (Jimerson, 1998). Apparently the poor schools needed the vouchers of the students with special needs for budgetary reasons. Based on his review, Henderson (1995) concluded that decentralization and privatization of the educational system was often associated with negative effects on students with special needs. Glascock, Robertson, and Coleman (1997) reported that charter schools faced many difficulties in financial management, dealing with social gaps and diversity, recruiting certified teachers, and treatment of students with special needs. These schools tended to overemphasize financial considerations. The emphasis on economic considerations may put the schools in a conflicting situation: on the one hand they need the vouchers and the public financial resources associated with the admittance of students with special needs; alternatively, accepting a significant number of these students can hamper the marketing efforts of the school since it can affect its image and prestige. Nathan (1997) pointed to the growing number of charter schools in the United States and to the high enrollment of minority students in these schools. Nathan's positive evaluation of the students' achievement, however, did not include any comment about students with special needs. One of the main requirements for establishing a charter school is the operation of systematic procedures of accountability. Accountability is a very complex issue when students with special needs are involved.

In spite of the inconsistent evaluations of the effect of privatization on students with special needs, certain findings indicated that parents' satisfaction from the education their children receive improved (e.g., Gorney & Ysseldyke, 1992). Parents reported higher levels of satisfaction, more involvement, higher academic achievements, and better responses to the special needs of the children. These are important findings even though they did not include objective measures of achievements. It was suggested that parents' satisfaction was based on factors other than academic achievement, such as the perceived social status of the child in the school, the stigmatization associated with his/her condition, and the sense of control the parents have on the child's education. This suggestion is supported by the finding that following the transfer of the child to the selected school, the categorical label of the child was often dropped and the special services to which he or she entitled stopped. Based on the available research it is difficult to conclude whether choice improved the academic achievements of regular students (Goldring et al., 1997) and of students with special needs.

Those who oppose an increase in parental choice suggested that choice has differential effects of various social groups (Jimerson, 1998). Jimerson argued that market economy and the increase in parental choice improves the situation of those parents and children who could use the newly opened opportunity more efficiently, and that their children get better educational services in the first place. Students from minority groups did not use these opportunities as efficiently as those of nonminority groups. Chen (1997) indicated that decentralized educational authorities resisted the need to invest adequate resources in students from lower socioeconomic backgrounds, minorities, and those with special needs. Reay and Ball (1997) proposed that increase of choice is a new social means by which social inequality and stratification are translated into educational inequality. It seems that the increase in choice and privatization and the decrease in the involvement of the educational authorities (e.g., the Ministry of Education) might worsen the situation of some of the special-needs students. This situation can exist despite increase in the number of services that can be selected and the increase in parental satisfaction. It is possible, then, that the advantages of choice and privatization are more pronounced in specific social groups but their advantage for other groups is questionable. Pijil and Dyson (1998) discussed the effects of changing special education financing and concluded that "the increase empowerment of parents as 'customers' does not necessarily lead to equity simply because different groups of parents are differentially equipped to take advantage of their new-found role" (p. 277). Even the stronger supporters of choice and free market organization of the schools were aware of the differential increase of parents' empowerment. Discussing regular education, Chubb and Moe (1997) acknowledged the limitations of the free market in advancing equality and therefore they recommended "an institutional structure in which market forces are carefully regulated" (p. 205). One of these regulations is that "all parents, but especially the poor parents, are to be assisted by public authorities in finding, evaluating, and applying to schools" (p. 25). It seems safe to conclude that unless a well-functioning procedure to assist parents and to regulate market forces is established, the results of individualization and privatization of the educational services might lead to an increase in the gaps among various social groups.

If it is assumed that similar processes operate within the population of D/HH students it may be concluded that only those parents who can effectively use the choices are going to benefit from the suggested changes. In other words, the differentiation within the population of D/HH students is going to increase according to socioeconomic lines. Socioeconomic background was previously found to have a stronger influence on the academic achievements of D/HH Israeli students than hearing ability, the presence of additional handicapping conditions, and intelligence (Weisel, 1989). It is, therefore, undesirable to further increase the gaps between various groups of D/HH students. Since the different sectors of the Israeli society differ with regard to socioeconomic status, the risk is that the gap between the general secular sector, the Arab sector, or the orthodox Jewish sector, and to a lesser degree the general religious Jewish sector, will increase. It is also likely that differences between central and peripheral geographical areas within each sector, and between poor and more affluent people within each sector will increase. This is a serious risk especially from the point of view of those who are concerned about the well-being of the less advantaged individuals in the society.

Two reservations about the previous discussion and conclusions that were made by the supporters of the change of the Israeli SEL should be noted. First, they argue that the increase in the gaps between various sectors and social groups is due to the improvement of the education of some of the students, but the situation of other students (those of relatively poor families) will not be necessarily worse. This is valid as long as choice is introduced in addition to the present available public services, institutions, and organizations. Furthermore, the supporters claim, the existing institutions and organization can handle the counseling and assistance needed for some of the parents. In addition, the existing institutions and organization can offer the necessary quality control needed for the services and to protect the interest of the students and their parents. These arguments of the supporters of the changes bring us back to the issue of excellence and equity in a zero sum game system that was discussed earlier. In addition, these arguments and suggestions put the existing public system in a conflicting situation since it will function as part of the system, by offering educational and rehabilitation services as well as a provider of counseling, quality control, and evaluation.

The second reservation that was made is that the consideration of the various groups within the D/HH population is relevant only if it is assumed that impaired hearing is a sufficient common denominator for having a coherent group of D/HH people in general. If hearing impairment is perceived as a characteristic of the individual, the effect of a change on "other" people with impaired hearing is hardly relevant. The significance of solidarity among the D/HH population, especially with regard to the social status and power of the D/HH people, to their struggle for fair rights and to their ability to actualize these rights was discussed earlier in this chapter.

SOME PRACTICAL CONSIDERATIONS

In this chapter an attempt was made to discuss several theoretical issues in the area of choice and privatization in the context of the Israeli educational system— all of which have ethical implications for the education of D/HH students. Three main characteristics of the Israeli educational system should be noted since they have clear influence on the feasibility of any change and on its outcomes: the small size of the population, the diversity of the population, and the sectorial organization of the educational system.

The number of students identified who have educationally significant hearing impairment in Israel is about 150 per year (Sela & Weisel, 1992). Although this is just a rough estimate, it indicates that the population of students is quite small. The general population and the population of D/HH people are also spread unevenly in the various regions of the country. About 54% of the population live in the three central parts of the country, Tel Aviv, Jerusalem, and the Central area (Statistical Abstract of Israel, 1999). The three other regions are relatively smaller. The educational system within each region is divided into the four main sectors of the Israeli society that were presented previously. The size of each sector varies from one region to another. This is especially pronounced with regard to the Arab sector. About 50% of this sector is in the north region of the country (Statistical Abstract of Israel). At present not every sector in every region offers special centers for the early education of D/HH children because of the limited number of students, the changes in the number of students from year to year, and the lack of professionals. Whenever parents are reluctant to send their D/HH child to a program or school outside their sector, the child is at risk for not getting proper educational services. Arab students find it difficult to attend Jewish programs and school because the spoken language they use, Arabic, is different from the language taught at school, usually Hebrew. Orthodox parents do not send their children to study in programs and schools of another sector for religious and cultural reasons. Practically this means that once the parent has chosen a sector the child can only participate in the programs that are available in that sector. Often that means that the educational service does not fit with the child's needs—for example, when there is no sign language environment offered to Deaf children in a specific sector (e.g., the orthodox sector). In this situation, it is not feasible to have alternative programs or centers or schools in each region and for each sector. Because of the size of the population and its cultural and religious diversity and because this diversity is accepted by the educational system in its sectorial organization, the number of alternative educational programs is limited, even for practical and financial reasons alone. At the most, the suggested changes of the Israeli SEL and the increase of alternative programs can be implemented in the general secular Jewish sector in the central regions only. The suggested change might, therefore, lead to a strong differential effect that will increase the gaps between various social groups along geographical and sectorial lines. Some will benefit. Many might lose.

CONCLUSIONS

The suggested changes of the Israeli SEL were initiated by a group of well-educated, relatively affluent parents and professionals who wanted their children to be educated by the AV approach that is not usually provided by the available educational centers. I can easily support their demand to have a choice with regard to their children's education, although I do not regard the specific approach they prefer as a recommended one. As a professional in the field of deaf education I object to the practice by which D/HH are isolated from other D/HH, and are associated with hearing peers only, even if this may enhance spoken language development (Weisel, 1991). This is because the isolation carries serious emotional, social, and psychological risks and might hamper the development of positive self-image and satisfying identity development. Such a practice of isolating D/HH from other children with similar conditions, which is based on the perception of deafness as an individualistic condition only, should be prevented, in my view, from becoming a mandatory and a universal practice or even the dominant one. Because it is possible, and even likely that increase in choice and privatization will cause more D/HH students to be mainstreamed and isolated from other similar children, it should not be accepted as the main basis of the educational policy. Privatization of the educational system of D/HH students involves serious risks to D/HH individual children as well as to the group of D/HH children and adults. The benefits are related to a relatively small group of D/HH students. Therefore, for principle and practical reasons the risks should be minimized even if as a result the freedom of choice of some D/HH student will be limited. If the results of the initiative to change the SEL will end up with formal and legal definitions of the rights of each individual student, with clear procedures by which the parents can ensure that every individual child is getting the educational and rehabilitation services to which he/she is entitled, with increases in the variety of methods and approaches that are provided by the existing public institutions and organization—all this will be a very big step forward. It is hoped that this can be accomplished without further hampering the solidarity within the deaf student population and within the society in general when the negotiations about the status of children and adults who are D/HH continue.

REFERENCES

Alexander, F. K. (1998). Vouchers in American education: Hard legal and policy lessons from higher education. *Journal of Education Finance, 24*(2), 153–178.

Antia, S. (1998). School and classroom characteristics that facilitate the social integration of Deaf and hard of hearing children. In A. Weisel (Ed.), *Issues unresolved: New perspectives on language and deaf education* (pp. 148–160). Washington, DC: Gallaudet University Press.

Arbeli, A. (2000, August 31). Parents' appeal to force the municipality of Beer-Sheva to allow students to attend schools outside the city was rejected. *Haaretz,* p. 2.

Bacharach, S. B. (1990). Putting it all together—educational reform: Making sense of it all. In S. B. Bachrach (Ed.), *Educational reform—making sense of it all* (pp. 415–430). Boston: Allyn & Bacon.

Barton, K. (1995). Disability: An issue for sociological analysis. In R. Kahane (Ed.), *Educational advancement and distributive justice—between equality and equity* (pp. 326–340). Jerusalem: Magnes Press.

Bat-Chava, Y. (1993). Antecedents of self-esteem of deaf people: A meta-analitic review. *Rehabiliation Psychology, 38*(4), 221–234.

Bunch, G. (1994). An interpretation of full inclusion. *American Annals of the Deaf, 139*(2), 150–152.

Chen, M. (1997). School choice as a bargain in a sectarian educational system. In R. Shapira & P. W. Cookson, Jr. (Eds.), *Autonomy and choice in context: An international perspective* (pp. 41–76). New York: Pergamon.

Chubb, J. E., & Moe, T. M. (1990). *Politics, markets, and America's schools.* Washington DC: The Brookings Institution.

Chubb, J. E., & Moe, T. M. (1997). Politics, markets, and equality in schools. In R. Shapira & P. W. Cookson, Jr. (Eds.), *Autonomy and choice in context: An international perspective* (pp. 203–248). New York: Pergamon.

Dunn, L. M. (1968). Special education for the mildly retarded—Is much of it justifiable? *Exceptional Children, 35,* 5–22.

Foster, S. (1989). Reflections of a group of deaf adults on their experiences in mainstream and residential school programs in the United States. *Disability, Handicap and Society, 4,* 37–56.

Fox, J. (1999). Sending public school students to private schools. *Policy Review, 93,* 25–29.

Gal, N. (1995). *The individual, the authority and the letter of the law—The Israeli supreme court's position on parent's choice of school.* Jerusalem: Research Institute for Innovation in Education, School of Education, the Hebrew University in Jerusalem (in Hebrew).

Glascock, P. C., Robertson, M., & Coleman, C. (1997). *Charter schools: A review of literature and an assessment of perception.* Paper presented the Annual Conference of Mid-South Educational Research Association. Memphis, TN.

Goldring, E., Hawley, W., Saffold, R., & Smrekar, C. (1997). Parental choice: Consequences for students, families and schools. In R. Shapira & P. W. Cookson, Jr. (Eds.), *Autonomy and choice in context: An international perspective* (pp. 353–388). New York: Pergamon.

Gorney, D. J., & Yesseldyke, J. E. (1992). *Students with disabilities use of various options to access alternative schools and learning centers.* Research Report No. 3. Enrollment options for students with disabilities. University of Minnesota, Minneapolis.

Henderson, R. A. (1995). Worldwide school reform movements and students with disabilities. *British Journal of Special Education, 22*(4), 148–151.

Inbar, D. (1994a). Choice in education in Israel. In D. Inbar (Ed.). *Choice in education in Israel—concepts, approaches and attitudes* (pp. 2–11). Jerusalem: The Ministry of Education (in Hebrew).

Jimerson, L. (1998). *Hidden consequences of school choice: Impact on programs, finances and accountability.* Paper presented at the Annual Meeting of the American Educational Research Association. San Diego, CA.

McGroarty, D. (1996). Bus ride to nowhere. *American Enterprise, 7*(5), 38–41.

Meyerson, A. (1999). A model of cultural leadership: The achievements of privately funded vouchers. *Policy Review, 93,* 20–24.

Nathan, J. (1997). Possibilities, problems, and progress: Early lessons from the charter movement. In R. Shapira & P. W. Cookson, Jr. (Eds.), *Autonomy and choice in context: An international perspective* (pp. 389–405). New York: Pergamon.

Paul, P. V., & Quigley, S. P. (1990). *Education and deafness.* New York: Longman.

Pijil, S., & Dyson, A. (1998). Funding special education: A three country study of demand oriented models. *Comparative Education, 34*(3), 61–79.

Reay, D., & Ball, S. (1997). "Spoilt for choice": The working classes and educational markets. *Oxford Review of Education.*

Schmid, H. (1986). The changing role of management in human services organizations. *Human Systems Management, 6,* 71–81.

Sela, I., & Weisel, A. (1992). *The Deaf community in Israel.* Tel Aviv, Israel: Association of the Deaf in Israel, National Insurance Institute, JDC Israel, Ministry of Labour and Social Affairs.

Shapira, R., Haymann, R., & Shavit, R. (1995). Autonomy as ethos, content as commodity: An Israeli model for controlled choice and autonomous schools. In R. Kahane (Ed.). *Educational advancement and distributive justice—between equality and equity* (pp. 358–374). Jerusalem: The Magnes Press, The Hebrew University.

Statistical Abstract of Israel. (1999). Jerusalem: Bureau of Statistics.

Stinson, M. S., & Lang, H. G. (1994). Full inclusion: A path for integration or isolation? *American Annals of the Deaf, 139*(2), 156–159.

Tucker, B. P. (1983). *Board of Education of the Hendrick Hundson Central School District v. Rowley:* Utter chaos. *Journal of Law and Education, 12*(2), 235–245.

Underwood, J. K., & Mead, J. F. (1995). *Legal aspects of special education and pupil services.* Boston: Allyn & Bacon.

Weisel. A. (1989). Educational placement of hearing impaired students as related to family characteristics, students' characteristics, and preschool intervention. *The Journal of Special Education, 23*(3), 303–312.

Weisel, A. (1991). Routes to postsecondary education for hearing impaired students in Israel. In E. G. Wolf-Schein & J. D. Schein (Eds.), *Postsecondary education for deaf students* (pp. 57–65). Edmonton, AB: Educational Psychology, University of Alberta.

Weisel, A. (1998). Unresolved issues in deaf education. In A. Weisel (Ed.), *Issues unresolved: New perspectives on language and deaf education* (pp. xvii–xxii). Washington, DC: Gallaudet University Press.

Willms, J. D., & Chen, M. (1989). The effect of ability grouping on ethnic achievement gap in Israeli elementary schools. *American Journal of Education, 97*(3), 237–257.

APPENDIX

Important or Main Points

- The early educational decisions for learning language at home may spur questions and disagreements when the child is to later attend a formal education program.

- It is at the start of preschool or school in Israel, like many other developed nations, that many ethically based judgments are formulated relative to placement and language of instruction.
- Pragmatically, educational options may be limited for financial reasons, small population, and lack of trained professionals. In addition, options may also be limited because of history, ideology, political will, religious/cultural affiliation, ethnic background, and gender roles.
- The individualistic versus societal perspective can and often has very different educational agendas. Any discussion about ethics and parental choice for placement is carried out within a certain social and political climate. This climate is reflected in the education policy of both regular and special education.
- Parents may not realize that the availability of program options, relative to method and language of instruction is often more limited than they were led to believe.
- Ethics and choice of placement is constantly changing. Change reflecting general social, political climates, and the educational climates of both regular and special education.
- Deafness perceived from medical/audiological perspective encourages the maximum level of integration of D/HH students with hearing students. A social perception supports the establishment of special educational settings—special schools or special classes for D/HH students.
- Parents may need to realize that placement decisions can reflect a trade-off between academic success and social-emotional variables for many children with hearing losses.
- The quality versus equity debate arising from sociopolitical orientation has very strong influences on the provision of educational services and educational placements for students with hearing impairments.

Follow-up References or Suggestions

- R. Shapira, R., & Cookson, P. W. Jr. (Eds.). (1997). *Autonomy and choice in context: An international perspective.* New York: Pergamon.

Ethical Questions for Consideration

- When considering educational placement, whose rights should prevail and in what order—the child's, the parents', the professional's, the opponent/support ad hoc group's, the government, or societies?
- Continuing on from the previous question—should there be a change in the prevailing rights with the age of child, the passing of time, population increases/decreases, political changes, social grouping, and such?

- Does the student placement or language of instruction or instructional program need to stay the same over the full period of a child's formal education? Is it even appropriate to think that it should?

7

EDUCATIONAL PLACEMENT

WENDY MCCRACKEN

AUTHOR INTRODUCTION

I am a Senior Lecturer in the Education of the Deaf at the University of Manchester, UK, where I am responsible for the training program for teachers of the deaf. Prior to working at the university I worked as a teacher of the deaf and educational audiologist. I have been fortunate to work in a wide range of settings, including preschool, nursery, primary, and secondary school settings, both as a class teacher and as a visiting teacher. I have a particular interest in early-years work, audiological management, and professional training for those working with deaf children.

A CASE TO CONSIDER

The local school is a busy, noisy working environment attended by all the kids in the neighborhood. Jake's parents are delighted that he seems to settle well, and his teacher of the deaf goes in twice a week to provide support and guidance. Jake finds it tough but has made some friends and is making progress albeit rather slow progress. The teacher of the deaf has mentioned that a special school for the deaf some distance away is having an open day and invites parents and Jake to join her there. Jake's parents have followed all the advice and attended all the clinic appointments. They have always trusted the visiting teacher of the deaf and were delighted when she helped them get a place for Jake in the local school.

Now the parents are faced with a new challenge. Jake has settled but is working well below his potential. He has made progress but this has been very slow and Jake is well behind his peers. Friendships are superficial and playground games seldom include him. The school is totally supportive but feel that Jake's real needs are no longer being met. Will a visit to the special school help to reassure parents that the local school is the right place? Will Jake, in the presence of deaf peers, show a side of his character as yet hidden? Will he want to leave his local friends for this new environment? Will he have to become a weekly boarder at the school? Jake's parents can't bear to think of him going away from home but do not want to deny him deaf friends and specialist intensive teaching. They have always believed in inclusive practice but wonder if inclusive can mean something other than their vision of the local school. Is there a right answer? Can Jake's present learning needs, emotional needs, and family needs be met elsewhere? Can the family maintain their close links with Jake at a distance? Will he lose contact with local friends? Will he feel at home with deaf peers? Is there a right answer?

INTRODUCTION

Education is an experience that families have in common. Parents, grandparents, and neighbors have all attended school. The type of education program, length of time within the school system, and curricular load will have varied. Memories of friends, particularly demanding teachers, favorite and least liked lessons, sports events, school plays, report forms represent a strong collective understanding of what education is about. For the majority of parents of children who are deaf, education is about the local neighborhood school. For deaf parents of deaf children, education is more likely to be about attending a school for the deaf outside the locality. Whatever experience provides a backdrop for parents to draw upon, it bears little relationship to current provision, present understanding of the learning process, curricular content, technological support, and methods of assessment. The diversity of learning needs among children who are deaf means that no single placement option will be suitable for all. No placement should be viewed as a final option rather that it is appropriate at a given point in development. Children's learning and personal needs change over time. Any educational placement has to be viewed as part of a larger educational program that should be flexible and responsive to individual needs.

In making choices about the educational placement of an individual deaf child, families are making decisions that will reverberate throughout the child's life. While teachers involved may be strong advocates of a particular approach, contact is relatively transitory. Families may seek to apportion blame for decisions made years earlier, and may regret not taking advice or following professional guidance more rigorously. Teachers may, as part of their professional development, modify or even change their views on what constitutes good educational practice. Ultimately the early years of family life are precious and any advice and support given should recognize this.

EARLY CONSIDERATIONS

Lewis (1999) points out that "many professionals express surprise that the parents of deaf babies are so quick to voice their anxieties over their child's schooling and job prospects." While parents expect many major changes in lifestyle with the arrival of a baby these changes are against a background of the "known" world. Considerations of educational placement, mode of communication, working with a range of professionals, technology, and specialist programs are not part of the expected package. Identification of deafness presents many challenges for parents who have no experiences to draw upon, no expectations to refer to, and often, no close family or personal friend to consult. Questions regarding schooling and employment cannot be placed within a known framework, nothing can be assumed.

Deaf Parents

For Deaf parents the situation may initially appear to be somewhat simpler. Such parents have an understanding, empathy, and knowledge of deafness. Personal experiences of education will provide a resource that can be drawn upon. Major changes in educational practice and legislation, however, challenge the accepted understanding of the nature of deaf education in the twenty-first century. The advent of cochlear implantation, legislative pressure for mainstreaming, introduction of sign bilingual programs within mainstream settings, use of learning support assistants, improvements in FM systems of amplification, the possibilities of digital amplification, the use of Individual Education Programs (IEPs) all mean that Deaf Education has changed. It has changed not only in terms of where it is located but also in how it is delivered and in the outcome measures used to gauge effectiveness. The expectations of Deaf parents may thus be very different from the educational provision available and from their own experiences of deaf education.

Initial Placement

Childhood is special for families and does not normally include an unknown adult being attached to the family or a young child being removed to educational provision "for their own good." Appointments, targets, IEPs, early-years curricula are not part of general family experience. Usually, educational placement for families of deaf children involves placement of a professional within the family setting. Although professionals supporting families of deaf children may be very welcome within families, they are not chosen by the family. These professionals, classically teachers of the deaf, are allotted a caseload. Some may be specialists in early-years work, whereas others may have a generic caseload or may teach in a specialist facility and be part of an outreach program. For individual families either their home becomes a counseling, support, or teaching area for at least part of each week, or families may have to travel to a facility that provides specialist input. Families have little choice in this matter, being subject to the local arrangements and provision. This initial placement of a professional within the family offers the potential for sensitive family-centered support but also presents many challenges. As specialists, teachers of the deaf are also "gatekeepers." Individual teachers of the deaf have both knowledge and usually personal experience of a range of educational options. Additionally teachers may, inappropriately, bring strongly held personal views to bear on families, either by failing to explain all the available options or by placing particular stress on one option to the detriment of others. Hearing parents are disadvantaged in having no personal or family experience to draw upon. Interestingly, in a recent review of good practice in deaf education undertaken within the UK (Powers et al., 1999) it was noted that: "Parents of young deaf children involved in this study reject a 'consumer model' in which a range of options is discussed with them, rather they are looking for consistency, commitment and a high level of professional expertise" (p. 216).

While professionals have moved to recognize the importance of a family-centered approach (NDCS, 1996) there is evidence that families want a clear and well-defined approach that professionals can deliver in a sensitive manner. Characteristically all the parents interviewed in the Good Practice Review (Powers et al., 1999) had been made aware of a range of communication options and types of educational placement available. The feature most valued was a strong, professionally informed teacher of the deaf who inspired confidence and who was actively involved in joint planning for the future. Such trust and dependence of the families of deaf children on teachers of the deaf places a responsibility on all those who have information to share this in an open nonpartisan way.

School Entry

The time at which children enter part-time or full-time educational provision varies considerably. It is hard to argue against any child being at home within the family unit for the early years of life. In the past young deaf children, yet to establish clear patterns of communication, have been removed from families and placed in special provision for deaf children. Such placements would, for many children, be at some considerable distance from home, be residential, and would effectively separate child from family. The lack of linguistic skills would make explanations difficult and severely restrict contact over distance. Children in this situation are likely to become institutionalized, taking meals in a larger more formal setting than at home, going on outings in a more formal group, having routines that reflect the need to run an efficient school rather than necessarily meet the needs of individual children. Such practice within the UK is now seen as outdated and inappropriate. All children have a range of needs—personal, social, and emotional as well as linguistic. Childhood should be secure and caring, based on a sense of trust and understanding between family and child. It is hard to imagine the justification for removing deaf children from their families in the early years of life.

THE POLITICAL FRAMEWORK OF PROVISION

The current legislative steer for mainstreaming or the inclusion of all children reflects a major international agreement on the rights of all children. In a 1994 UNESCO conference in Salamanca, delegates called upon all governments to "adopt as a matter of law or policy the principle of inclusive education, enrolling children in regular schools unless there are compelling reasons for doing otherwise" (UNESCO, 1994).

An interesting caveat was included in the Salamanca declaration. This specifically mentioned the special learning needs of deaf and deaf/blind children as being different from other disability groups.

> Educational policies should take account of individual differences and situations. The importance of sign language as the medium of communication among the deaf, for example, should be recognized and provision made to ensure that all deaf persons have access to education in their national sign language. Owing to the particular communication needs of deaf and deaf/blind persons, their education may be more suitably provided in special schools or special classes and units within mainstream schools. (UNSECO, 1994a, p. 18)

In asserting the right of "all deaf children" to have access to the curriculum through the medium of sign language UNESCO fails to take into account a number of ethical issues that face families and professionals alike. The term "deaf" left undefined, encompasses a heterogeneous population of individuals. Such individuals may have any degree of permanent childhood deafness, and will vary considerably according to causes of deafness, age of onset, age of identification, age of amplification. Each child, in addition to being deaf, will also have a personality, a range of hopes and dreams—as do their parents—that demand an individual approach. Medical models of deafness are frequently criticized because they "emphasize what a person cannot do (or cannot do as a hearing person would)" (Reagan, 1990, p. 74). However, the learning needs of children with mild to moderate hearing losses are dissimilar to other children with severe or profound degrees of hearing loss. Placing all deaf children together as a group with similar needs fails to take account of the diverse nature of this group and the diverse family situations involved.

Communication Mode

It is well established that the majority of deaf children have hearing parents who are unlikely to have any knowledge of deafness or sign language other than that gleaned from the media (Moores, 1996). It is equally well established that sign languages are fully-fledged linguistic forms which have all the subtlety and richness of spoken languages (Sutton-Spense & Woll, 1999). Within the UK it is largely a matter of geographical accident whether a family is offered support in developing sign language skills. This raises major ethical considerations. Families of deaf children rely on local service providers to supply information regarding mode of communication, educational placement options, and audiological support. If a particular education authority, responsible for the provision of local educational services, has a specific policy—oral, sign-bilingual, or total communication—families realistically have little choice. It is now practice within the UK that families have the right to be given information regarding all modes of communication. This does not translate into all options being locally available. Rather, the low incidence of permanent childhood deafness makes it practically impossible to have all educational options within the locality. For many parents of deaf children the choices of placement are stark, either the local mainstream school or placement outside the immediate community. The degree of flexibility and ability to provide individually tailored educational placements and support packages in local schools are heavily dependent on the degree of urbanization and economic prosperity. For those deaf children living in rural areas the educational choices are reduced. Local educational provision in urban areas is more likely to have experience in meeting a wide range of educational needs and in the provision of a range of educational options.

Lack of previous experience of deafness may, however, result in low educational expectations, inexperienced management of audiological equipment, and lack of deaf awareness, all of which could compromise the situation of a deaf child. It should not be assumed that lack of experience is necessarily negative. With the support of qualified teachers of the deaf, in person, by facsimile, e-mail, or videoconferencing, local mainsteam staff can be invaluable. For some families choice is an inappropriate description of the process of education placement. Families opting for a sign-bilingual education face a relatively limited selection of provision. It is possible to find such provision in some mainstream schools but this option is unusual. Usually children will need to attend residential provision at a distance from the home community.

Inclusion

The term "inclusion" has many definitions and within these there are contradictions. To be more than integration a concept of inclusion must encompass social, linguistic, emotional, and cultural inclusion. For deaf children inclusion is a multifaced concept. Within the UK it is estimated that 85% of deaf children are being educated within a mainstream setting (Lynas, Lewis, & Hopwood, 1997). Location of a child within a mainstream setting is simple. Ensuring effective inclusion with curricular access at an appropriate level, with peers both in class and in the playground, and ensuring a growing sense of identity and personal responsibility for the individual deaf child is, however, a complex and demanding task. Families of deaf children and professionals are faced with a polemic situation. Does inclusion mean the local neighborhood school or the school where a child is linguistically, cognitively, and socially supported, which may be a school for the deaf? Conversely can a child sent to residential school for the deaf really be part of the neighborhood? Attempts to promote and secure inclusive education may take many forms and pose a series of challenging questions.

Individual Support

In some mainstream settings individual children are pre-and post-tutored. Such support involves a teacher of the deaf working in close harmony with mainstream staff to identify the most appropriate time to provide such support. Individual deaf children are provided with a highly structured session that may address specific aspects of the curriculum or, for older pupils, may provide a time to address issues relating to personal development. Pure inclusionists would argue that this type of support excludes children from the mainstream of educational experience and in doing so stigmatizes them. Such political correctness fails to take into account the effect of deafness on the acquisition of spoken language, room acoustics, the limitations of amplification, and the need to ensure that all children with a hearing loss are cognitively engaged with the curriculum rather than being passive recipients. It is important to allow older children to be active partners in support programs:

> Pupils have a say in their own support programs. They can negotiate the amount of support they receive and up to a point the subject(s) they omit from the curriculum in order to receive support—they can elect to have "support" as one of their curricular options. Support teachers by class teachers rely heavily on the comments and feedback offered by the pupil, and pupils are encouraged to take responsibility for their own learning needs from as early an age as possible. (Powers et al., 1999, p. 91)

In contrast to this approach, mainstreaming for some deaf children is concerned that the individual child is located and supported within the mainstream class. Such support may be provided by a number of professionals including teachers of the deaf, learning support assistants, and communication support assistants. In-class support takes many forms and involves a range of staff. The principle of providing a facilitators to help to ensure curricular access on behalf of an individual deaf child is uncontroversial. The placement of an additional adult within the classroom raises a number of questions. What is the exact role of this additional adult? Does the child seek clarification of a concept through this adult or the class teacher? How does the child cognitively access the curriculum? Do learning support assistants have the knowledge and skills base to support all aspects of the curriculum? Are children allowed to make mistakes and to learn from them? Can children be over-supported and lose a sense of independence and personal worth? What happens outside of the classroom at play and dinnertime? What are the effects of having an adult attached to an individual child for a major part of the school day? Research into this aspect of deaf education suggests that there is awareness of the problem of over-supporting and that more focus is now being placed on the introduction of independent learning skills (Powers et al., 1999, p. 96). It would appear that the addition of in-class staff may be helpful but only if this is planned for and the potential problems are identified and dealt with before such support is provided. The aim should always be for children to develop skills that permit them to learn independently both in respect of the curriculum and in respect of the wider social environment of the school.

Pragmatic Perspective

Inclusion is a concept that intellectuals may debate at length but to which families often bring a pragmatic perspective. Families have a basic objective that is unrelated to educational provision per se; the basic objective of families is to have healthy and happy children who grow into healthy and happy adults. Different families' understanding of exactly what this entails will be distinct and in some cases may be hard for professionals to understand. Inclusion for families will often reflect the everyday experience of childhood—going to the local store, learning to swim, joining in at birthday parties, taking part in social, cultural, and religious ceremonies with the rest of the family group.

For professionals involved in deaf educational provision, inclusion is a controversial concept. It may be argued that inclusion for a deaf child is only meaningful if it is with deaf peers. In a review of good practice in deaf education undertaken within the UK it was noted that, "the importance of discrete, specialized provision is seen as entirely compatible with the goal and or practice of inclusion" (Powers et al., 1999, p. 79). Both oral and sign-bilingual schools for the deaf shared a belief in the importance of inclusion within wider society as a goal for all deaf children and viewed separatist provision as supporting rather than undermining inclusive practice. For the majority of Deaf adults inclusive practice falls outside their range of experience. Rather than seeing mainstreaming of deaf children as a social and political aim that will ensure an equal place in society many feel that inclusion is a denial of the basic rights of the individual. Mainstreaming may be viewed as assimilation of deaf children into hearing society, denying them access to Deaf culture (British Deaf Association, 1996). A range of approaches has been developed to enable mainstreamed deaf children to have access to Deaf culture. This may not be as easily achieved in more remote areas where there are no other deaf children or adults. In this case the residential family weekends can help to ensure that this important aspect of a child's personal development is not overlooked. Pure oralists may find this a contentious issue but have also to bear in mind that, however successful any child with permanent deafness is, he/she will grow up to be a deaf adult. Children find difference interesting. Deaf children have a considerable benefit in meeting and sharing experiences with Deaf adults. It is adults who find the concept of Deaf culture challenging. Access to deaf role models should be enriching for all concerned. The tacit assumption, however, that because someone is deaf they are a suitable role model for deaf children is clearly unacceptable. Anyone working with and influencing children should be appropriately vetted and trained irrespective of their hearing status.

LEGISLATIVE FRAMEWORK

The legislative framework, within which education is provided, seeks to provide basic rights and to establish the responsibilities that national and local governments have to ensure that all children have equal access to education. The reality is that in the majority of situations either political realism or cynicism tempers altruistic goals. The scope and mandatory requirements of such laws vary but governments have a vested interest to ensure that as many of the population as possible will develop to their full potential and become independent economic units that contribute to society. In pursuing this goal governments both at national and local level have fixed budgets. The focus is generally on the bigger picture, putting minority areas, such as education of the deaf, relatively low on the list of priorities. Laws governing the provision of education for deaf children are generally considered within the remit of special education. At present within the UK, Local Education Authorities have to provide mainstream education for children with special educational needs, provided that the provision is appropriate to the identified individual needs of the child. Such placement must be demonstrated to be the most efficient use of resources and compatible with the efficient education of other children.

The Mainstream

The educational possibilities available to any family are largely an accident of geography. To understand the range of possibilities, current practice in the UK is used to exemplify the range and variety of provision available at present to families. Situations will be very different in other parts of the world. Families are, however, entitled to be made aware of the diversity of approaches and placements options available; without such knowledge the possibility of real discussion and debate with professionals is severely contrained. The dilemmas faced by many families are similar. For each type of provision basic information relating to organization, potential benefits, and drawbacks are illustrated. The individuality and innovative practice that can be illustrated in any school should be borne in mind. The majority of children with permanent childhood deafness in the UK are educated within the mainstream of education, most usually within their local neighborhood school.

One major consideration is the withdrawal of deaf children into individual or small group work situations. A balance has to be achieved to ensure deaf children have cognitive and linguistic access to the curriculum. The opportunity to provide a small group situation outside the noise and bustle of the mainstream classroom appears to have considerable benefits for all. The deaf child is not isolated, a group of children can benefit from intensive work, children can be encouraged to tackle work colaboratively, make best use of amplification systems, consider complexities of class work away from the stresses of mainstream education. The choice of who goes out with the deaf child is problematic. Depending on the criteria used to choose children to be withdrawn for group work, deaf children may well be working with children who have learning disability, specific reading disability, or behavior problems rather than children of a similar cognitive ability. This compromise is far from ideal; it may support the work of the class teacher and provide quality time for a larger group of children, but it is unlikely to be optimum provision for a deaf child. Figure 7.1 outlines the elements of the child being educated in the local school.

There is a high degree of flexibility within individual education authorities. One example is an oral setting where individually mainstreamed deaf children meet with other deaf pupils and deaf adults on a regular basis. A deaf teacher of the deaf working with hearing colleagues introduces all deaf children to sign language. In addition a program of personal and social development is run to provide an empathetic setting for the discussion of sensitive issues. The IEP is used to develop personal support packages for all pupils. Teachers of the deaf work in close cooperation with mainstream teachers in joint planning and assessment. Support is provided to individual deaf children in the form of pre- or post-tutoring by a teacher of the deaf on a withdrawal basis. In other mainstream settings the

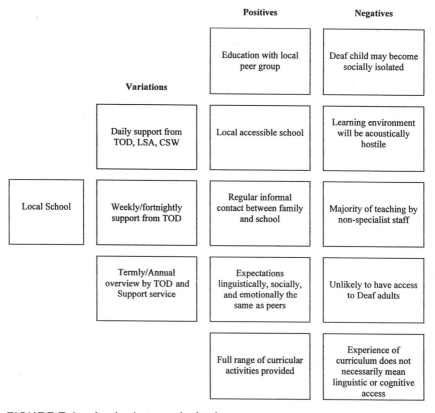

FIGURE 7.1.   Local mainstream school option.

majority of support may be in-class and may be undertaken by Learning Support Assistants (LSAs). The majority of support may come from unqualified staff. Typically, LSAs will have received in-service training and will work under the direction of a teacher of the deaf. Responsibilities, however, may vary considerably. Expectations of those staff may not be commensurate with pay, with the job description, or with the status held within the school setting.

Resource Base or Unit

Specialist resource bases or units are attached to a mainstream school or college. Such bases may employ a single teacher of the deaf or a team of teachers of the deaf. The resource base may function as the main teaching area for a group of deaf children or may be a resource that provides pre- and post-tutoring to a group of deaf children, together or individually. Deaf children may be on the roll of a mainstream teacher or on a separate resource base roll. There is considerable diversity of provision; some of the possible arrangements are illustrated in Figure 7.2.

No single unit or resource base will operate in exactly the same way. As pupils pass through the system different needs will be met in a number of ways. The availability of a teacher of the deaf in situ mean that high levels of support can be provided when the need arises. It is important, however, that such flexibility arises from student need rather than availability of qualified staff. Individual pupils can develop independent study skills with the knowledge that the teacher of the deaf is a point of referral. The presence of other deaf children provides a sense of community and may provide an important base for identity resolution in the teenage years. It is important that the deaf pupils move between two groups, their hearing peers in the mainstream class and their deaf peers in the unit or resource base. In doing this pupils are provided with a small window on the world, where the existence of multiple communities between which people constantly move, is illustrated.

A Deaf Perspective

In considering educational placements, the British Deaf Association (BDA) asserts that in the case of a resourced mainstream school or unit, "there should be a minimum number of deaf pupils in each year group and in each resourced support" (BDA, 1996). Such a statement fails to take into account the low incidence of permanent childhood deafness. In order to achieve such groupings deaf children would have no option but to travel, in many cases considerable distances in order to be educated with their deaf peers.

Special School Settings

Day and residential schools for the deaf were the first type of provision generally available for the deaf children. Such schools have evolved to provide a highly specialized option for a minority of deaf children. Inevitably such schools will, for the majority, mean residential placement away from home. Specialist staff and

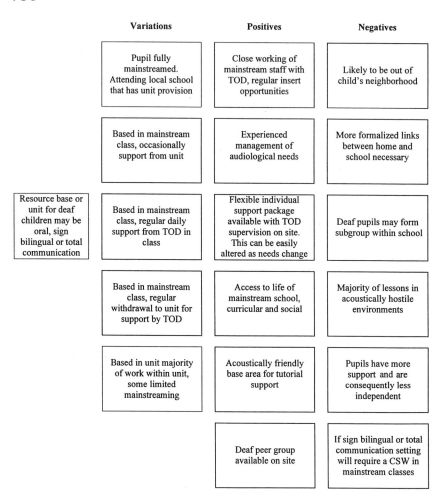

Variations	Positives	Negatives
Pupil fully mainstreamed. Attending local school that has unit provision	Close working of mainstream staff with TOD, regular insert opportunities	Likely to be out of child's neighborhood
Based in mainstream class, occasionally support from unit	Experienced management of audiological needs	More formalized links between home and school necessary
Based in mainstream class, regular daily support from TOD in class	Flexible individual support package available with TOD supervision on site. This can be easily altered as needs change	Deaf pupils may form subgroup within school
Based in mainstream class, regular withdrawal to unit for support by TOD	Access to life of mainstream school, curricular and social	Majority of lessons in acoustically hostile environments
Based in unit majority of work within unit, some limited mainstreaming	Acoustically friendly base area for tutorial support	Pupils have more support and are consequently less independent
	Deaf peer group available on site	If sign bilingual or total communication setting will require a CSW in mainstream classes

Resource base or unit for deaf children may be oral, sign bilingual or total communication

FIGURE 7.2.   Resource base or unit provision.

facilities together with the availability of small class groups, a deaf peer group, and high levels of support ensure such schools are, while declining in number, still an important part of the educational provision available. It is unlikely that such provision will be lost altogether, the diversity of learning needs among deaf children suggest that there will always be schools for the deaf. The role fulfilled by such schools is likely to become increasingly specialized.

Schools for the deaf have changed radically in the past two decades, partly in a response to the move to mainstreaming and partly in response to changes in the knowledge and skills base. See Figure 7.3 for a summary of the components of specialized day and residential schools for the deaf. Many such schools meet the challenge of isolationism by having planned mainstreaming programs that

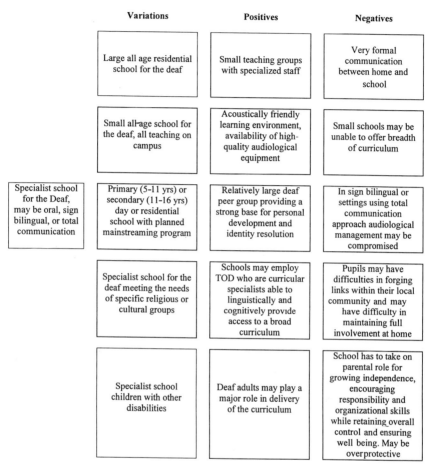

	Variations	Positives	Negatives
	Large all age residential school for the deaf	Small teaching groups with specialized staff	Very formal communication between home and school
	Small all-age school for the deaf, all teaching on campus	Acoustically friendly learning environment, availability of high-quality audiological equipment	Small schools may be unable to offer breadth of curriculum
Specialist school for the Deaf, may be oral, sign bilingual, or total communication	Primary (5-11 yrs) or secondary (11-16 yrs) day or residential school with planned mainstreaming program	Relatively large deaf peer group providing a strong base for personal development and identity resolution	In sign bilingual or settings using total communication approach audiological management may be compromised
	Specialist school for the deaf meeting the needs of specific religious or cultural groups	Schools may employ TOD who are curricular specialists able to linguistically and cognitively provide access to a broad curriculum	Pupils may have difficulties in forging links within their local community and may have difficulty in maintaining full involvement at home
	Specialist school children with other disabilities	Deaf adults may play a major role in delivery of the curriculum	School has to take on parental role for growing independence, encouraging responsibility and organizational skills while retaining overall control and ensuring well being. May be overprotective

FIGURE 7.3.   Day and residential schools for the deaf.

encourage links with local provision and the wider hearing community. Schools for the deaf within the UK have developed provision for more particular learning needs—for example, deaf children with disabilities, those choosing a sign bilingual approach, and deaf children with social and emotional difficulties.

Support for Learning

Whatever the placement available for children with permanent childhood deafness it is reasonable for families to assume that teachers trained to work with deaf children will feature prominently; this may be as class teacher, as a resource based teacher, or as part of a visiting teacher program. Within the UK such a specialist teacher would undertake second-tier training following initial training as a teacher.

Qualified teachers of the deaf have specialist skills in promoting the development of communication skills, helping to support linguistic and cognitive access to the curriculum, audiological management, and advocating on behalf of the needs of deaf children within their caseload. The majority of teachers working with deaf children are qualified and experienced professionals. However, in a survey of educational provision for deaf children in England the number of unqualified teachers working within deaf education was 246 full-time equivalents. Of these unqualified teachers 113 work within schools for the deaf, 107 within resource base or units, and 26 within mainstream (Eatough, 2000). Of greater concern is the total of 69 full-time equivalent teachers who do not intend to undertake specialized training. Families may assume that schools and services for deaf children employ only fully qualified teachers of the deaf. Within England and Wales teachers working within schools for the deaf or resource bases must qualify within 3 years of commencing work. This means that for some children a high proportion of their time within specialist provision may be with untrained teachers.

Lewis (1999) draws attention to a parent's disappointment and loss of confidence when she realized her child had been taught for 3 years by a teacher-in-training who failed to qualify and subsequently left the school. While parents have every right to expect that teachers are qualified to work within mainstream education this is not recognized in law within the UK. Once a child is identified as having special learning needs the right to have a suitably qualified specialized teacher is not protected by law. Present consideration of the qualification to teach deaf children within England and Wales by the Teacher Training Agency may help to address this problem (TTA, 1999). Parents should be aware that working within deaf education may not equate with qualified to work within deaf education.

FAMILY FRIENDLY SERVICES?

Families are in the unusual position of having to rely on professional advice regarding educational placement. Those involved within deaf education often have strongly held views not only about what educational placement is appropriate but also about what the objectives of education are for an individual child. Such views and opinions have potentially, a very strong influence on family decisions. For families the effects of such influences are permanent. As families become increasingly aware of the options, the challenges that each option brings and the contradictory advice emanating from "professionals" and a range of interested parties complicates their situation. As one parent of a boy deafened by meningitis eloquently noted:

> It was a strange time, three weeks or four weeks before we'd had a little boy now we had an officially deaf child... People came round and said "this is the new game off you go." (McCracken & Sutherland, 1981, p. 143)

A Practical Approach

One education authority considering the potential for staff over influencing families produced a booklet for parents. This included a range of points for parents to help focus on the suitability of a school for a child with special needs. It is used to encourage parents to ask themselves and others a series of questions to help inform their choice (Powers et al., 1999, p. 164). The situation of individual teachers of the deaf requires a broad perspective, the knowledge of the full range of current provision, and great sensitivity. A highly specialized school for the deaf may offer the potential of academic achievement but may also be a very expensive option raising the concerns of the local authority, or may be at a considerable distance from home, raising major concerns within the family. Similarly, a local mainstream setting may offer ease of access and close contact with family and the neighborhood, but may not be able to offer adequate levels of individual support needed by a particular child. A change in school personnel may result in changes in the quality of provision offered. A teacher of the deaf aware of this situation has to make a moral decision whether to discuss his or her reservations. To discuss such reservations would be to impugn the professional integrity of a colleague but in not discussing such reservations a teacher would be undermining the trust of a family. By arranging visits to a range of provision it may be possible to allow families to identify particular strengths and weaknesses. For those families where the choice is very limited as a result of geographical location the situation is more problematic.

Resources for Families

For families the objective is likely to be based on a finding school situation that meets the individual needs of their child and one in which their child can be an active participant. For others the objective may be ideological or political. A potential glut of information is now readily available for families from voluntary agencies, charitable sources, and via the Internet. Many agencies that ostensibly work on behalf of deaf people provide a bewildering array of contradictory information for families of deaf children. Such information may help to inform families and enable them to make the most effective use of educational services provided or challenge outdated or ill-informed professional practice. Alternatively, it may well entrench families into feeling that the field of deafness is a political battlefield in which they are casualties. Information relating to mode of communication is one of the key areas that families will seek advice on. Decisions regarding choice of communication mode has a direct effect on choice of educational placement. The following are examples of information provided in resource packages aimed at the families of deaf children:

- "The deaf child's ability to learn to listen will be adversely affected by the use of sign or over use of gesture." (DELTA, 1999)

- "Without Cued Speech I would not have been able to get as far as I am now and would have faced many more barriers in the hearing world." Quote from Rachel, a profoundly deaf, UK, B.Sc. (Hons) Graduate member of the Institute of Physics, presently employed as a microwave engineer. (Cued Speech, 2000)
- "The British Deaf Association believes that bilingualism represents the most appropriate form of education for the majority of Deaf students. Bilingual education is an approach which uses both the sign language of the Deaf community and the written spoken language of the hearing community." (BDA, 1996)

For families pondering the most appropriate educational placement for their deaf child the potential for confusion is significant. It may be more useful to consider the evidence based on academic achievements in deaf children and to balance these against the hopes of families rather than the political comments of interested parties. The fact, however, that such an evidence base is both complex and incomplete offers little comfort to parents making placement decisions. A review of the educational achievements of deaf children considering data from British and American research (Powers, Gregory, & Thoutenhoofd, 1998) provides a starting point. The end result for families of deaf children is that decisions made regarding placement can only reflect what is reasonably available, that the Local Education Authority (LEA), federal, or state authorities will agree to provide or fund or what the family is able to afford. The cost of going against local provision may be considerable in both financial and emotional terms. While school education is free to all within the UK and LEAs have to fund "out of area provision" for those children for whom they are unable to offer an appropriate education, this is not true elsewhere. The emotional cost to a family of choosing to send a child away from home can be considerable. This may result in a deaf child being placed locally within the mainstream school beyond a point that is reasonable. Parents must be able to rely on professionals to offer them impartial advice, to have the opportunities to visit a range of settings, and most important the chance to talk to other families of deaf children from a range of settings. This is relatively easy in an urban setting but far less so in an isolated rural setting. Parents can become very strong and opinionated advocates of particular educational settings or approaches. Is it appropriate for teachers of the deaf to point this out to less experienced parents or does this in itself devalue the trust that parents place in professional opinions?

The Role of Deaf Adults

Deaf adults are increasingly becoming involved within the field of deaf education, as teachers of the deaf, educational psychologists, communication support workers, preschool consultants, and learning support assistants. A major challenge is to ensure that appropriate training and development is provided for this group.

Within the UK all those wishing to become a teacher of the deaf must complete initial training within the context of mainstream education prior to specialist training. This requirement places a considerable barrier in the way of some Deaf candidates. Training, within the UK context, of other Deaf professionals working within education is less well defined. Some individual education authorities have introduced both induction and training schemes. The need to establish nationally recognized training routes that ensure knowledge, understanding, and skills are at an appropriate level, is pressing. Because audiological status is not an indicator of fitness for purpose, all hearing and Deaf adults should have appropriate training, which includes detailed skills assessment prior to working within deaf education.

The low incidence of deafness and stereotypic portrayal of deaf adults within the media together with societal attitudes, mean that the majority of hearing families have little experience of deafness. The referral point for many will be aging grandparents with acquired hearing loss. Families face the challenge of trying to visualize their child's future with at best a poorly informed model of what this might look like. The most gifted and experienced hearing teacher of the deaf has much to offer but cannot talk "from the inside," from practical experience.

Home Setting

A project run within the UK established an early intervention program that sought to address these issues (Sutherland & Kyle, 1993). Deaf consultants worked in close collaboration with hearing teachers of the deaf. The intervention package included weekly support from a Deaf consultant, a separate visit from a teacher of the deaf, and weekly attendance at a preschool parents group. The Deaf consultants had a number of roles, acting as a role model for the family, introducing or improving signing skills, and to be a Deaf friend to the family (Sutherland & Kyle, 1993).

> All three groups (families, teachers of the deaf, and Deaf consultants) agreed that one of the most effective elements of the intervention programs had been to address parents' anxieties over not understanding what is meant for their child to be deaf. (Young, 1999, p. 162)

Within this project the training needs of the Deaf consultants were clearly identified and met prior to program commencement. Furthermore, detailed research of the impact of the program on families has been undertaken. The relationship between families and the Deaf consultants did promote a clearer understanding of Deaf experience, but also created a problem. "Parents were confronted with the realization that there were things that a Deaf person knew about deaf children because they were Deaf, that they as parents could not know about their own child" (Young, 1999, p. 163). One parent, in response to Young's analysis, drew attention to the conflicts that can be introduced to families by positive Deaf role models. Canavan notes "it puts pressure on parents to hide their true feelings" (Canavan, 1998, cited by Young, 1999, p. 175). Although those Deaf adults within the project were highly motivated, trained, and committed to providing a quality service it is inappropriate to assume that the Deaf community at large will have a particular interest in the needs of the families of deaf children.

Self-Esteem

Throughout all educational provision for deaf children, whether fully mainstreamed or in highly specialized provision outside the mainstream, one of the primary objectives of education is to enable individuals to develop their full potential and become an independent adult. In order to function successfully, deaf children, like all children, have to develop positive self-esteem. This can begin in the Nursery setting. One example of such an approach is cited by Powers et al. (1999),

> The nursery provides an interesting example of the formation of positive deaf identity at a very early age. The strength of the model is perceived to be a nursery designed primarily for deaf children where deaf children outnumber hearing children, yet in a mainstream school. By this arrangement the children are helped to realize that they are deaf but being deaf is not odd. In this way they can develop a positive deaf identity prior to entering formal schooling. (p. 143)

It is not only within such specialist settings, unavailable to the majority of deaf infants, that positive self-esteem is promoted. For individually mainstreamed deaf children regular meetings with deaf peers can be arranged and positively promoted through a range of activities. An exciting opportunity to promote positive self-esteem and a deaf identity is via the Internet where a specialist secure site has been launched to promote "better literacy and communication for deaf and hearing children at home and at schools worldwide" (Deafax Trust, 2000). As part of the site a deaf role-models section is included and all those visiting the site are invited to nominate their deaf hero. The opportunities for deaf children to have access to positive deaf role-models and a deaf peer group has thus moved beyond what can be offered within the immediate environment.

In-Class Support

For deaf children in mainstream settings a range of professionals may be involved in providing daily in-class support. Such support may be in oral, sign-bilingual, or Total Communication settings. The demands made upon deaf children in mainstream classes are considerable not only because of poor acoustics, distance, poor lighting, and the distractions that characterize groups of young children, but also because of the linguistic and cognitive demands made of the class. A support worker can help to facilitate an individual deaf child's access to the curriculum but the way in which this is done varies and has considerable implications for the individual child. In many respects sign language support in class is easier and less disruptive than in an oral setting. The lack of competing auditory signal means that the class teacher and hearing peers will not be disturbed. Those providing such support should be proficient in sign language, be familiar with the curriculum area being covered, and be able to work with groups of children as well as the individual deaf child. The question of what "proficient" in sign language means is less well established. In the United States a growing acceptance and expectation that educational interpreters will be working within mainstream educational settings have matched the rise in inclusive practice. Moores (1996) cites a report that identified in excess of 500 educational programs that employ interpreters. The lack of training opportunities for those sign language interpreters working within educational settings is problematic. The needs of children are very different form those of Deaf adults. Training for interpreters focuses on adult situations, particularly within the fields of medical and legal interpreting and not on delivery of the curriculum. The ability of class teachers to make the most effective use of interpreters has received little attention (Beaver, Hayes, & Luetke-Stahlman, 1995).

DEAF CHILDREN WITH DISABILITIES

There is a group of children with permanent childhood deafness who have other disabilities. This group is diverse and complex. Lack of internationally agreed terminology compromises attempts by researchers to provide a strong evidence base. There are specific subgroups for whom highly specialized educational placement has been developed, for example those identified as deafblind. For the majority of children with permanent childhood deafness who have other disabilities, provision is limited. Placement may be within the mainstream of education, within a specialist resource base, within a specialized school setting other than a school for the deaf, or within a hospital setting. Access to support services for deaf children is restricted by a variety of factors including: sensitive audiological assessment of need, identification of special learning needs when compounded by hearing loss, and attitudes limiting access to support services. When educational services for deaf children are limited, services may be faced with a stark choice. If limited by economic or staffing factors, should support go to a child who with that support can gain recognized attainment points or to a child who is likely to require considerable help throughout life? It is self-evident that both children have the same right to sensitive efficient support. A major challenge is to ensure that all children have access to appropriate assessment of learning needs and that this assessment should be formative, identifying a starting point. The limitation of audiological assessments will mean that teachers of the deaf have a very important role to play in audiological profiling of children with severe and profound cognitive impairments, to ensure that any educational provision takes into account sensory status when planning programs.

The growing evidence base identifies a number of facts that must be taken into account when planning provision, considering placements and support packages. Incidence of disability co-occurring with deafness is high. Table 7.1 summarizes recent studies of children with hearing impairments that were concerned with identifying the incidence of other educationally relevant disabilities.

The lack of specialized training opportunities for teachers of the deaf working with this complex group of children together with the pressures of time and caseloads led to some marginalization of this group. The need to establish the value-added component related to the cost of the provision of additional support time is challenging. Teachers of the deaf may need to work on a regular

TABLE 7.1   Recent Studies Identifying the Incidence of Educational Relevant Disabilities of Children with Hearing Impairments

Study	Overall Incidence
Karchmer, 1985	31%
Schildroth & Motto, 1994	34%
Stredler-Brown & Yoshinago-Itano, 1994	41%
Fortnum et al., 1996	39%

basis, providing individual support to a child, family, or classroom teacher, provide input to a multi-professional team or act as the bridge between health and educational services. Families may be unaware of the specialist help that is available, may be encouraged to see sensory loss as low priority within a hierarchy of special needs, or may prefer to focus on other aspects of individual needs rather than hearing loss. As mainstreaming ensures that an increasingly diverse group of learners are within the mainstream of education it is likely that teachers of deaf children with additional disabilities will have increasing demands made on their time for support in planning and delivering services for this group of learners.

OUTCOME MEASURES

In the past the degree of hearing loss identified has been used as a strong indicator of the type of educational placement that should be considered for an individual child. Within this model degree of hearing loss, a two-dimensional measure of what cannot be heard, would be the primary factor in deciding type of educational placement. Children with a profound hearing loss would be educated separately from those with a severe or moderate hearing loss. Such an approach is no longer tenable. Research evidence suggests that degree of hearing loss is a poor predictor of educational attainment (Powers et al., 1998). A wide range of factors relating to the individual child, the family, the type of placement, the level, quality and consistency of support available needs to be taken into account. In a small-scale research program considering the outcomes of mainstream education for deaf pupils (Lewis & Hostler, 1998) focused specifically on children with severe or profound degree of hearing loss educated within a natural aural approach. All subjects were prelingually deaf with an average hearing loss of 95dBHL in the better ear. This group of subjects attained examination results that were above the national average, the median reading age for the group was 14.6 years with 28% at or above the ceiling of the test (16 years). Measures regarding speech intelligibility, social participation, and levels of satisfaction with support were all rated very highly. The key factor identified as significant was the quality and consistency of the educational approach, underpinned by rigorous audiological management. It is axiomatic that the outcomes of any educational placement are likely to be strongly influenced by the level of skills available and the degree of rigor with which these are applied.

CONCLUSIONS

Placement is about the whole child, their family, friends, acquaintances, and the hopes and dreams of parents and their child. It is not about political correctness, but it is about what people want to be the end product of education. The "best" educational placement for any child is always a compromise, what is actually available and what we want, all are constrained by geography, some economically, some linguistically, some by religion or culture. Families want the "best" but the concept of best is varied and may conflict with professionals' view of optimum or even good. Nothing is fixed—children are adaptable and will, often against the odds, demonstrate their skills, likes, dislikes, worries, and joys. As families grow together adjustments are made to changing needs, both real and perceived. The support of families, whatever the family is in the context of an individual child, are central to that child's development. No individual placement exists that will meet all a child's needs. A strong and involved family is the most important aspect of any child, helping to guide, support, and to accept each individual for what they are.

REFERENCES

Beaver, D. L., Hayes, P. L., & Luetke-Stahlman, B. (1995). In-service trends: General education on teachers working with educational interpreters. *American Annals of the Deaf, 140*(1), 38–42.

British Deaf Association (BDA). (1996). *The right to be equal: The British Deaf Association Education Policy.* London: British Deaf Association.

Cued Speech. (2000). *Information sheet.* Cued Speech Association.

Deafax Trust. (2000). *Deafchild International.* Presentation at the 19th International Congress on the Education of the Deaf, Sydney, July 2000.

DELTA. (1999). *DELTA's Education Policy: The right to be heard.* DETLA.

Eatough, M. (2000, May). Deaf children and teachers of the deaf, Raw data from the BATOD Survey 1998. *BATOD magazine.*

Fortnum, H., Davis, A., Butler, A., & Stevens, J. (1996). *Health service implications of changes in aetiology and referral patterns of hearing impaired children in Trent 1985–1993. Report to Trent Health.* Nottingham and Sheffield: MRC Institute of Hearing Research and Trent Health.

Karchmer, M. A. (1985). A demographic perspective. In E. Cherow, N. Matkin, & R. Trybus (Eds.), *Hearing impaired children and youth with developmental disabilities: An interdisciplinary foundation for service* (pp. 36–56). Washington, DC: Gallaudet College Press.

Lewis, S. (1999). Educational routes-ways, and means. In J. Stokes (Ed.), *Hearing impaired infants: Support in the first eighteen months* (pp. 163–191). London: Whurr.

Lewis, S., & Hostler, M. (1998). *Some outcomes of mainstream education.* London: Ewing Foundation.

Lynas, W., Lewis, S., & Hopwood, V. (1997). Supporting the education of deaf children in mainstream schools. *Journal British Association of Teachers of the Deaf, 21*(2), 41–45.

McCracken, W., & Sutherland, H. (1981). *Deafability not disability.* Clevedon, UK: Multilingual Matters.

Moores, D. F. (1996). *Educating the deaf: Psychology, principles, and practices* (4th ed.). Boston: Houghton Mifflin.

National Deaf Children's Society. (1996). *Quality standards in pediatric audiology, Vol. 2.* London, NDCS.

Powers, S., Gregory, S., Lynas, W., McCracken, W., Watson, L., Boulton, A., & Harris, D. (1999). *A review of good practice in deaf education.* London: RNID.

Powers, S., Gregory, S., & Thoutenhoofd, E. (1998). *The educational achievements of deaf children.* London: Department of Education and Employment, HMSO.

Reagan, T. (1990). Cultural considerations in the education of deaf children. In D. Moores & K. Meadow-Orlans (Eds.), *Educational and developmental aspects of deafness* (pp. 73–84). Washington, DC: Gallaudet University Press.

Schildroth, A., & Motto, S. (1994). Inclusion or exclusion? *American Annals of the Deaf, 139*(2), 163–171.

Stredler-Brown, A., & Yoshinaga-Itano, C. (1994). F.A.M.I.L.Y. assessment: A multidisciplinary evaluation tool. In J. Rousch & N. D. Matkin (Eds.), *Infants and toddlers with hearing loss: Family-centered assessment and intervention* (pp. 133–161). Baltimore: York.

Sutherland, H., & Kyle, J. (1993). *Deaf children at home: Final report.* Bristol, UK: Center for Deaf Studies.

Sutton-Spence, R., & Woll, B. (1999). *The linguistics of British Sign Language: An introduction.* Cambridge: Cambridge University Press.

Teacher Training Agency. (1999). *National specialist educational needs specialist standards.* London: Teacher Training Agency.

UNESCO. (1994). *The Salamanca statement and framework for action on special needs education.* World Conference on Special Needs Education: Access and Quality, Salamanca, Spain, June 7–10, 1994.

UNESCO. (1994a). *The standard rules on the equalisation of opportunities for persons with disabilities.* New York: UN Department of Public Information.

Young, A. (1999). Hearing parents: Adjustment to a deaf child—The impact of a cultural linguistic model of deafness. *Journal of Social Work Practice, 13*(2), 157–176.

APPENDIX

Important or Main Points

- After the difficult and complex early decisions about amplification, language, and communication, educational placement is probably the consideration that looms largest in the minds of those concerned with the education of children with hearing losses.

- It is unfortunate, but an education decision is one that parents and guardians must make while both their child and their knowledge about deafness are at a tender age. Hearing parents appear to be particularly disadvantaged—knowing little about deafness, but even for deaf parents much has changed since their early educational experiences.

- The decision makers must consider the best interests of the child, but temper that with reality and circumstances that have ethical aspects. The most valued feature for parents was a strong, professionally informed teacher of the deaf who inspired confidence and who was actively involved in joint planning for the future.

- The multifaceted concept of "inclusion" is a complex goal for children with hearing losses. Attempts to promote and secure inclusive education may take many forms and pose a series of challenging questions.
- Although individual support is usually acknowledged as a necessary educational component for a child with a hearing loss, there may be drawbacks and negative concerns as well depending on approach and extent of provision.
- Provision of educational services may take many forms: mainstream, resource base or unit, special schools.
- Providing "family-friendly" services should be a goal when the educational placement of students with hearing loss is the consideration. This service includes resources, acknowledging the role of deaf adults, building self-esteem, and providing support.
- The educational placement for students with deafness and other disabilities is even more complex than just a single disability.

Follow-up References or Suggestions

- UNESCO. (1995). Special needs education: Access and quality: Issues and viewpoints from the Salamanca debate [Videorecording].
- Although dated for some information and focused on legislation in the United States, there is still useful information on topics such as legal rights, educational options, least restrictive environment, due process, and such in Nix, G. W. (Ed.). (1978). *The rights of hearing-impaired children.* Washington, DC: A. G. Bell Association for the Deaf.
- The "Mainstream Placement Question/Check List" by Gary W. Nix is still a useful guide in examining the major parameters contributing to a successful mainstream placement. (See Nix, 1978, p. 345–346)

Ethical Questions for Consideration

- Should the young deaf child be exposed to more assessment—this time to clarify placement?
- Does early intervention rob the child of a childhood?
- Is the least restrictive environment, those settings commonly held in high regard—the neighborhood school, the integrated preschool—actually the least restrictive environment for the child with a hearing loss?
- Does the integrated placement meet the requirements of providing like-companions, a variety of role models, or both hearing and deaf teachers who bring different strengths?
- Archbold (2000) questioned whether cochlear implants influence the educational decisions beyond "How" and "Where"? Will the decision concern only educational placement? Will the CI then restrict the choices over time if it becomes obvious that changes should be made because of the child's lack

of progress? Will the implant shift the decision-making responsibility over the long term to that of the educator?

- Special or mainstream school—does the child have access to a variety of sign users, both children and adults, during the day in order to sustain language growth?
- Is it possible to deliver the curriculum in sign? Consider: Baker in Lynas (1999) asks, "are these 'practical problems to be overcome rather than problems of principle that are insurmountable,' or will the scale of difficulty defeat the bilingual purpose?" Personally, watching education in general, I don't believe the resources that many hope for will be available.

8

CURRICULUM
CONSIDERATIONS

GREGORY R. LEIGH

AUTHOR INTRODUCTION

I commenced my career in teaching deaf students at the Queensland School for the Deaf in Brisbane, Australia, and have subsequently held positions as a teacher, teacher-in-charge, itinerant teacher, and curriculum consultant in a range of rural and metropolitan locations in Queensland. For most of the last 15 years I have worked in teacher education and research in three Australian states. In 1999 I was appointed Assistant Chief Executive (Educational Services) at the Royal Institute for Deaf and Blind Children in Sydney and Conjoint Associate Professor of Special Education at the University of Newcastle, Australia.

My professional qualifications include degrees in Education and Special Education from Griffith University in Brisbane, a Master of Science in Speech and Hearing degree from Washington University in St. Louis, and a PhD in Special Education from Monash University in Melbourne.

My current position affords me the opportunity to remain active in university teaching, research, and publication. Importantly, however, my position provides me with a significant role in the process of curriculum development for deaf and hard of hearing students. I remain committed to the view that curricula must be genuinely reflective of, and responsive to, students' specific situations. In this chapter I seek to broadly define the notions of "curriculum" and "situation" with a view toward underlining the importance of a process that aims to consider all of the possibly relevant issues and perspectives in the design of curriculum for students in this group.

CASES TO CONSIDER—SUI MAY AND JENNY

Sui May is 3$^1/_2$ years of age and, with her parents Wendy and Kwong, is enrolled in a home-based early intervention program for deaf children and their families. The program operates on a family-centered philosophy and aims to provide parents with the necessary information and support for a wide range of potential communication options. The program further aims to assist parents in making the necessary choices associated with future preschool and school education for their children.

Sui May is profoundly deaf but has some usable amplified hearing in the speech range. The family has been involved in the program for more than 2 years and maintains a commitment to the development of Sui May's auditory–oral communication skills. Although English is their second language, both parents are committed to Sui May learning English as her first language. The decision to pursue an oral approach was, however, less than clear-cut since her aided audiogram suggests that Sui May gains little benefit from the modern high-powered hearing aids that she has worn since she was 14 months of age. She was assessed as a candidate for cochlear implantation when she was 2 years of age but was found to have a significant retro-cochlear component to her hearing impairment with very poor prospect of significant benefit from such a device.

Over the last 6 months it has become increasingly obvious to Sui May's home-support teacher that her oral communication skills are not developing as effectively as would be desired. Her speech and language skills are not commensurate with those of either her hearing-age peers or her peers with similar degrees of hearing impairment.

Sui May's parents experience difficulty with both written and spoken English. Her father is a blue-collar worker who labors long hours to sustain the family income. Her mother also works outside the home (although only part-time), and has difficulty in keeping the schedule of home visit appointments. Both are caring parents but their work commitments and language difficulties have meant that the interaction and communication practice that is required for successful development of language skills is often difficult to sustain at home. Both parents and the extended family have struggled with Sui May's hearing impairment and still tend to deny its significance on the basis of their belief that the development of spoken skills is only a matter of time.

Because Sui May is now past her third birthday, the time has come for the commencement of a transition process to preschool education. Sui May's parents have the option to seek her enrollment in any one of three alternative reverse integration preschool programs: (1) an auditory-oral preschool, (2) a Total Communication preschool, or (3) a sign-bilingual (English/Sign Language) preschool.

Sui May's support teacher, Roslyn, is personally very strongly committed to oral educational approaches but is aware that there is a strong likelihood that Sui May will not develop the necessary spoken language skills to benefit from a preschool program which is based entirely on oral communication. This view is more firmly held by the program's speech pathologist who believes that Sui May shows a genuine disposition to visual communication.

Enrollment in a preschool that is based on the use of signed communication (either a sign-bilingual or Total Communication program) will require a commitment to the learning and use of sign language or a sign system that is unlikely to be viable for Sui May's parents. Equally, however, the commitment to home support of an oral language and speech development program is likely to be problematic for the reasons already outlined.

The issues that need to be considered in making the first and most fundamental curriculum decision in planning Sui May's school education are far from being unidimensional. There is a myriad of issues to be considered and a range of individual perspectives to be adopted and appreciated. What mode of communication is most likely to provide for a mutually fulfilling relationship between Sui May and her family (including her extended family)? What mode of communication is likely to produce maximal access to the important learning experiences that should be part of any preschool curriculum? Can effective educational outcomes be achieved if the chosen language is only able to be supported at school and how will this affect the quality of both her school and home learning and living environments? Are these decisions that should be made entirely by Sui May's parents? In the context of curriculum development and implementation should parental decisions about communication approach be incontestable elements of the subsequent curriculum process? If not, then what should be the evidentiary standard for challenging (or overruling) such decisions? Is it possible to offer sufficiently high standards of evidence to support alternative curriculum decisions where issues such as communication mode and program location are concerned?

Jenny is a teacher in a day school for deaf children. The school has operated on a Total Communication philosophy for many years but has recently been slowly including the use of natural sign language in preference to simultaneous communication in speech and manually coded English. The school's curriculum is purported to follow the regular state-accredited curriculum guidelines for children in regular schools. Class teachers are, however, afforded considerable freedom and flexibility in curriculum design and implementation—particularly at the level of individual class teachers' decisions about curriculum objectives and content.

Jenny is responsible for a class of seven 8-year-old students. Like most teachers in the school, Jenny maintains a strong commitment to the development of her pupils' English language skills and focuses considerable resources (i.e., time on task, texts, and materials) on this curriculum area. Nevertheless, her pupils' English language skills remain significantly below age-appropriate standards in regard to written English language ability.

Over a period of years of similar focus of attention, there has been a systematic lack of emphasis on outcomes in a number of other core curriculum areas—particularly in mathematics and social sciences. The parents of Jenny's pupils are well aware of their children's levels of English language skill. They are, however, somewhat less informed as to the gap between the age and grade level for their children's performances in other curriculum areas. Over time, individual teachers have acknowledged in both program planning and reporting that there is an expectation of some academic delay in these areas commensurate with delays in language development.

State-sponsored achievement testing is arranged for all students in all schools (regular and special) at strategic points (Grades 3 and 5) to assess both collective and individual outcomes against core curriculum standards. Although participation in these testing programs is mandated for all children in regular schools, registered special schools for children with disabilities can elect not to participate in the program. Classes at the Grade 3 and Grade 5 level at Jenny's school do not routinely participate in the core curriculum standards assessment program. This is justified on the basis that the alternate curriculum programs followed by students in the school dictate a different rate of progress through the curriculum to that expected in the mainstream. It is argued that the testing regime that is applied according to age level is not a fair or accurate measure of progress against the school-based objectives pursued in those curriculum areas. The assessment that is conducted within the school in the nonlanguage curriculum areas indicates that there is an age-grade gap between student outcomes and core curriculum outcomes that widens as the students progress through the school. In other words, the students fall progressively farther behind age level expectations as they progress through the school.

Jenny, like other teachers in the school, has the capacity to set alternative curriculum parameters for her students. Jenny feels compelled to pursue this course of modified curriculum expectation for two reasons. First, she believes that there are more immediate and important curriculum priorities in the area of language and literacy. And second, there is too great a gap between current levels of performance and grade level to be able to redress the discrepancy in the context of the available time and staffing resources.

Jenny's dilemma is one that ensues, at least in part, from a series of curriculum decisions taken at previous points in time. Individually each decision may or may not have been well considered. Regardless of degree of diligence, however, those decisions have clearly had a considerable cumulative impact on the academic performance outcomes for the students concerned. From an ethical perspective, several issues should concern us here. There is the obvious question of whether such outcomes are a reasonable reflection of the reality of the learning situation and potential of Jenny's students or whether such outcomes are more a consequence of other factors that were more susceptible to control. It may be, for example, that the disappointing student outcomes are the progressive consequence of locally planned curricula that were too narrow in scope because they were unnecessarily isolated from available curriculum guidelines and monitoring processess. Such an explanation would clearly be cause for great concern. Of even greater ethical concern, however, is the possibility that the cumulative gap is a consequence of either (a) insufficiently high expectation of performance of the pupils themselves, or (b) the setting of unduly conservative objectives because of previous teachers' concerns about being held accountable for lack of performance against those criteria.

INTRODUCTION

The dilemmas that confront Roslyn (Sui May's support teacher) and Sui May's family in the first scenario, and Jenny in the second scenario, concern decision making. Their decisions and the educational processes that will be set in motion by those decisions are all part of the complex process of curriculum design, modification, and implementation.

Curriculum development is fundamentally a process of effective and informed decision making. The decisions involved in curriculum development and implementation are all made in a particular social context and are inherently value-laden. In this chapter we will examine the premise that truly effective curriculum development requires that educators approach the process as concerned, well-informed, and ethical decision makers who place the highest priority on the rights and dignity of the deaf or hard of hearing students that they serve in making those decisions.

DEFINING CURRICULUM

The word "curriculum" is used constantly by educators and all those with an interest in education but is frequently not subject to high levels of mutual understanding of its meaning. In popular usage, the term is used alternatively in broad and narrow terms. For some purposes, curriculum is seen broadly as being "what happens in schools." For other purposes, people view curriculum as being specifically the content of the syllabus that dictates certain teaching and learning processes and content in schools.

The former definition is too broad—although probably only marginally so. Clearly, much that happens in schools and other educational facilities and programs falls outside the realm of curriculum. The activities of the gardener or the use of the school as a community meeting venue are clearly not part of the curriculum. Most other activities, however, can be seen to be part of the curriculum process. The latter definition is certainly too narrow. The curriculum must be considered as more than the mere concept of a syllabus—much more than a narrow collection of subject headings with predetermined learning objectives and experiences. Curriculum refers not only to courses of study or defined lists of learning experiences but to the effects on student learning and development of an extremely wide set of arrangements. These arrangements include variables such as staffing policy, teaching strategies and styles, school/program organization, and assessment and reporting procedures. Very broadly then, it can be argued that "curriculum" refers to:

> [. . .] all the arrangements that a school (or other educational program) makes for student's learning and development. It includes the content of courses, all student activities, teaching approaches and decisions on the facilities provided and the ways in which teachers and classes are organized. (Education Department of Victoria, 1985, p. 9)

Such a definition serves to highlight the fact that any curriculum is inherently an expression of values. The communities served by schools (and other such educational programs and facilities) may not easily reach agreement about these values. In most societies there are some beliefs held in common but there is also much that can differentiate individuals and groups of individuals that can serve to make curriculum decisions controversial. Further, there is considerable potential for some of the values that underpin curricula to be unstated and taken for granted. There is clearly the potential for a school's curriculum to be based, at least in part, on a set of assumptions and behavior patterns that are not consciously articulated but nevertheless reflect the values of the majority (or an influential minority). It is this potential, or reality, that has given rise to the concept of the "hidden curriculum."

The "Hidden" Curriculum

The concept of an ever-present hidden curriculum is one that has been described by numerous authors (Jackson, 1968; Seddon, 1983). Variously, authors have examined this phenomenon and concluded that "…formal listings of areas of knowledge and ordered beliefs inevitably fail to indicate fully what is both taught and learned in a school" (Claydon, Knight, & Rado, 1977, p. 33). In other words, what we set out to do, the so-called official or planned curriculum, accounts for only some of the learning outcomes for children and other participants in the curriculum process. Desirably, there is much additional learning that is the unplanned consequence of our planned arrangements. The hidden curriculum does not refer to this outcome but rather to the unplanned learning that is a consequence of our unplanned arrangements.

The field of education for deaf and hard of hearing children is fertile ground for the existence of such hidden curricula. To illustrate this point, it is appropriate to return briefly to the hypothetical early education program of Sui May in our opening scenario. Families encountering this program for the first time are setting out on a voyage of discovery with open-ended outcomes. The parents' aim, and the aim of the program, is for them to make a choice about both communication mode and educational approach for their child. It is the educators' aim and desire to be supportive of that choice and to provide the necessary support to enable that choice to be effectively implemented.

While families are endeavoring to make a choice about future communication mode and educational options they will be susceptible to a range of both intentional and unintentional learning experiences. Teachers and other consultant professionals will undoubtedly provide them with a range of planned information and learning experiences related to a variety of educational placement and communication options. However, the attitudes of those professionals toward the various types of communication, their own relative abilities to use those options, and their comfort and ease in relating to children and adults who use those forms of communication will all be part of a rich set of learning experiences for the families. Although probably unintentional, messages about the various options—both positive and negative—will be inevitably and effortlessly learned. To the extent that particular professionals are unenthusiastic about or incapable of using a particular communication option comfortably, the more effectively an element of a hidden curriculum will have been constructed.

In schools, the messages inherent in particular statements and actions of teachers are also seemingly effortlessly learned by children. This is particularly true for issues relating to cultural diversity and tolerance. Still, there is clearly a considerable potential for an influential hidden curriculum in early intervention programs and other early educational programs for deaf children where the "learners" are just as much the parents and the families of those children. The likelihood families will be susceptible to unintentional learning experiences as much as to the planned experiences is increased by the fact that they typically come to the task with no relevant background or experience relating to deafness. Almost every experience is a new and highly salient event with no prior knowledge to act as a filter or modifier of the information they receive.

Claydon et al. (1977) have argued that "no school can decide not to have a hidden curriculum. However, the content of the hidden curriculum in any one instance need not be left to blind chance" (p. 20). From an ethical perspective, the acknowledgment of the existence of this phenomenon necessitates that teachers and other related professionals involved in curriculum development for deaf children strenuously defend against the creation of a hidden curriculum that is contrary to the content of the planned curriculum. To pursue the current example, teachers in the first scenario with Sui May clearly must guard against the development of a hidden curriculum that provides an inherent bias toward a particular choice of communication mode if the stated curriculum calls for facilitation of family decision making through family-centered support.

The existence and potential power of the hidden curriculum is perhaps easier to conceptualize in the context of a classroom where teachers are continually communicating attitudes and assumptions through their actions and other behavior—albeit that they are often unaware or only partially aware of these behaviors and associated attitudes themselves. Often these attitudes are not so much their own as those of their social group, or even their professional group. Regardless of their origin, they become part of the learning experiences of students in that situation.

Clearly, curriculum is a wide-ranging concept that includes both official and hidden components and outcomes. These concepts must form part of our overall working definition of curriculum and warrant careful consideration from the perspective of ethical practice. Guarding against the development of a hidden curriculum requires a process of careful and complete disclosure and consideration of the issues and perspectives that relate to the particular situation. We will return to this issue later.

Official and Unofficial Curriculum

Returning to our earlier definition, it is apparent that the overall process of curriculum development involves an extremely broad set of decisions about an equally broad set of arrangements for students' learning. Such diverse curriculum decisions about all manner of arrangements ultimately give rise to an official cur-riculum—a set of shared understandings, if not specific and clearly stated school/program policies and procedures, aims and objectives, and strategies for achieving learning outcomes across a range of domains.

We have already noted the potential for discrepancy between these policies and the hidden curriculum that can arise as a consequence of the unwitting intrusion of values and attitudes into the process. The gap between stated cur-riculum and reality may, however, be much more deliberate in origin. As Bell and Pitt (1976) have noted, the mismatch may be the result of a teacher's refusal to operate within the bounds of curriculum parameters. Such refusal may stem from a perception that the stated curriculum aims and strategies are inconsistent with his or her own values and educational beliefs. Alternatively, Bell and Pitt noted that the lack of congruence between the official curriculum and particular practice of a teacher or teachers may be the result of more basic issues such as laziness, inefficiency, incompetence, or simply an inability to meet overly ambitious aims that have been incorporated into the official curriculum. It may also be a "deliberate and pretentious disguising of curriculum reality" (p. 10) in order to impress or appease someone or some authority including, for example, higher administrative authorities, parents of current or potential students, other teachers or schools, and so on. Regardless of the reason for the mismatch, the effect of the mismatch is to create a gap between the "official" curriculum and the "actual" curriculum.

The gradual process of devolution of curriculum authority to schools (Brady, 1990) could be seen to have made the likelihood of an official/actual curriculum gap less likely. There is, however, little evidence that such gaps have ceased to exist. Indeed, in the case of curriculum in schools for deaf students, where there has tradi-tionally been considerable curriculum freedom granted by education authorities, the potential for such a gap to exist remains significant. This is often evidenced in a gap between the grade-level description applied to groups of deaf students and the actual curriculum level being pursued in one or more academic subject areas by their teachers. Such a situation is not of ethical concern because of the alternate or amended nature of the curriculum being implemented but, as in the case of our sec-ond example scenario, because of the way that the situation is often portrayed to— or allowed to be perceived by—parents, and even the students themselves, as being age/grade appropriate.

CURRICULUM DEVELOPMENT AND IMPLEMENTATION IN PRACTICE

To return to our earlier discussion, it is clear that we are best served by a broad rather than a narrow definition of curriculum. If curriculum refers to all of the arrangements that are made for students' learning and development, then curricu-lum planning is a task of considerable dimensions. It is a process that involves participation by a diverse group of stakeholders that must collectively consider a wide range of matters. These matters include issues as diverse as staffing considerations and the organization of the built environment.

As broad as the range of potential "arrangements" may be, it remains the case that there are certain inescapable core curriculum arrangements which must be made—certain curriculum questions that must be addressed as a matter of course in any curriculum development process. When planning and organizing a curriculum for any school or other educational service for deaf or hard of hearing students, particular attention would appear to be warranted to at least the following fundamental curriculum variables:

- The establishment, organization, and statement of the aims and objectives of the school or service;
- The design of teaching and learning experiences to meet those objectives (acknowledging the need to design experiences that are inclusive of all learners, including those from different cultures and those with different abilities and/or disabilities);
- The organization of those experiences to ensure continuity across the years of schooling (Preschool-12);
- The assessment and reporting of students' progress as a measure of the achievement of the curriculum objectives;

There is certainly nothing new in this statement of issues for consideration. Tyler, as early as 1949, identified these issues and stated them even more succinctly as four questions that are fundamental to the curriculum design process:

- What educational purposes should the school seek to attain?
- What educational experiences can be provided that are likely to attain these purposes?
- How can these educational experiences be effectively organized?
- How can we determine whether these purposes are being attained?

This simplification of the core elements of the curriculum process is consistent with what is commonly called the "objectives" model of curriculum development but has also been variously termed the "rational," "logical," or "means-ends" model (Brady, 1990, p. 58). It is acknowledged that several alternatives have been proposed to describe the curriculum development process. For the most part, however, alternative models all acknowledge the importance of these component questions but suggest different (nonsequential) patterns of relationship among them. For our purposes, the significant issue here is not one of order but rather how effectively these questions are addressed and whether the process is conducted with a consistent view toward the best interests of all concerned. Stated another way, the issue that should concern us is whether curriculum development is undertaken within the context of well-informed and ethical decision-making processes—both individually and collectively (i.e., as a school or service). This raises the question of what it means to be personally or collectively ethical in decision making.

Ethics in Decision Making

There is no simple answer to the question of what it means to be ethical in the context of curriculum decision making. Ladd (1980) has argued that ethics "is an open-ended, critical and reflective intellectual activity" and to seek to specify it, as in formal codes of ethics for particular purposes, "is to confuse ethics with law-making" (p. 154). Others disagree and for this reason, codes of ethics for professional conduct are frequently controversial documents. Given this controversy, it is probably inappropriate to suggest any single "code of professional ethics" for curriculum design and implementation for deaf and hard of hearing students. Nevertheless, there is much in the literature on professional codes of ethics that can offer us some general guidance in responding to the question of what it means to act ethically in curriculum design and development.

The Center for the Study of Ethics in the Professions (CSEP) at the Illinois Institute of Technology began collecting codes of professional ethics more than 20 years ago. With the advent of the World Wide Web and with the assistance of the National Science Foundation the CSEP have made their collection available on-line (see http://csep.iit.edu/codes). Scrutiny of the many codes they have collected provides an opportunity to identify the principles that are commonly considered to be important in defining ethical practice. The principles that are common to many, if not most, of the codes governing professional practice in education and other cognate professions have been summarized in the six points listed in Figure 8.1. (Note: No organizations of teachers of the deaf are listed in the CSEP collection.)

Clearly, based on this list of principles, being ethical in curriculum decisions demands a high level of commitment to the well-being and advancement of the students being served. In addition, it demands a high level of commitment to the society that the students will become a part of, and a commitment to high standards of professional preparation and ongoing development of professional knowledge and skills. In particular, effective and ethical decisions demand a high level of knowledge and understanding of the specific curriculum development context or "situation."

In the remainder of this chapter we will briefly consider, as examples, some of the curriculum development questions as raised by Tyler (1949) from the perspective of the dictates of these general principles for ethical practice in decision making.

ADDRESSING CURRICULUM QUESTIONS
ETHICALLY—AN EXAMPLE

The first of the four curriculum questions raised by Tyler (1949) related to the establishment of objectives. In the context of this brief chapter, this first question provides a useful example to consider the range of ethical considerations that may be raised in the curriculum development process.

- **Nonmaleficence:** Often stated simply as "above all do no harm," this is probably the most often-stated principle in codes of professional ethics in the helping professions. It refers simply to the notion that professionals should not make any decision or take any action that will likely occasion any negative outcome for those being served.

- **Beneficence:** The concept of seeking to do good, of being proactive, and alert to all opportunities to advance the welfare of those being served.

- **Justice:** The concept that all individuals should be treated with fairness and equity. Where different treatment or opportunities are offered, this principle dictates that this should be by virtue of a clear and appropriate rationale.

- **Competence:** Often stated as the need for due diligence, this principle encompasses the notion that professionals should make decisions and take actions on the basis of the highest standards of professional competence and with the utmost of care. As often stated, this principle dictates that professionals comply with relevant regulations in regard to minimum standards for preparation and accreditation and often also dictates the need for ongoing professional development.

- **Recognition of limitations:** The notion that all professionals should be aware of the limits of their ability and expertise and should operate within those limits. This principle dictates that, when the limits of knowledge or expertise are likely to be exceeded, the practitioner should refer to, or enlist the assistance of, other professionals.

- **Value awareness:** The notion that there be a genuine and concerted effort to understand and take account of the various value structures that may be in play—particularly in regard to how those values may differ from both mainstream social values and the values of the individual or overall organization delivering the service.

FIGURE 8.1. List of principles common among codes of professional conduct in education and cognate professional fields.

Bunch (1987) suggested that, according to the particular perspective that is adopted, the curriculum objectives identified for deaf or hard of hearing students may be (a) the same as those applicable to children in mainstream schools, (b) an adaptation of those applicable to mainstream schools and services, or (c) a completely alternative version of the objectives applicable in regular education programs.

Moores (1990) noted that there has been a history of specialized curriculum objectives being considered both necessary and appropriate for students who are deaf. In the early days of special educational provision such alternative curricula often focused on industrial and vocational rather than academic outcomes—particularly in residential schools for the deaf. Historically, however, the main curriculum priorities in education of the deaf have been in the areas of speech reception and production and the mastery of the grammar of the local spoken language. In this regard, Moores noted that teacher-training programs have traditionally emphasized these areas over the academic areas of mathematics, science, and the social sciences. The automatic acceptance of alternative nonacademic curriculum objectives for deaf students, however, is now much less common. Nevertheless, there remain strong arguments as to why alternative curriculum objectives, and associated curriculum provisions, are not only desirable but also necessary in certain circumstances for deaf and hard of hearing students.

The point of emphasis here should be on the concept of "specific circumstance." There can be little ethical defense possible for a position which suggests that all students with impaired hearing should, as a consequence of that fact alone, have educational objectives that differ from those for any other student in the society at large. The notion of a "one size fits all" approach to implementation of specific curriculum objectives for deaf and hard of hearing students has rightly given way to an approach based on response to individual learning needs and circumstances. The notion of individualized programming is now commonplace in educational theory and practice and seeks to make the curriculum responsive to the specific educational program requirements of individual students.

This principle of individualization of programming is one that has considerable support. In the context of educational provision in the United States, for example, this principle is enshrined in law through the Individuals with Disabilities Act (IDEA). Originally enacted by Congress in 1975 as the Education for all Handicapped Children Act (commonly referred to as Public Law 94-142), the law dictates that any child with a disability should receive educational and related services that are designed to meet their unique needs through the development of an Individualized Education Program (IEP). Whether dictated by law or simply by sound pedagogical practice, the principle of individualization obviously can give rise to a wide range of different curriculum development outcomes where deaf and hard of hearing children are concerned. The breadth of those alternative outcomes depends on the choices and decisions about objectives made by those involved in the curriculum development process.

It is important to recognize that in many places the process of individualizing curricula for deaf or hard of hearing students sits alongside existing processes for designing and implementing curricula (i.e., processes that operate for all students at the local level and at the level of central educational authorities). In Australia, as elsewhere, there are guidelines for the content of "core" curriculum components imposed by the state. Although schools are afforded some flexibility, a centrally administered process dictates many core objectives.

Ethically, there would appear to be little debate that, for children for whom hearing impairment is their only educationally distinguishing characteristic, there should be no question of routinely choosing to eschew the curriculum objectives that would apply to any other student. Few people who have either knowledge or direct experience of deafness, however, would deny that there are certain characteristics of deaf learners that may necessitate the inclusion of some objectives that differ from those for hearing learners. For deaf students then, the process of individualization is one of determining whether there are additional educational objectives that should be met as a basis for achieving the core objectives of regular education, and/or whether there are additional specific objectives that relate to their status as a deaf person (e.g., objectives that may relate to their need for support in developing language and communication skills or to their particular social and cultural needs).

From the perspective of ethical decision making, the process seems straight-forward. Those responsible for curriculum design and implementation are charged with the responsibility of making ethical decisions about alternate or additional curriculum objectives based on considered analysis of individual students' particular educational needs. This task, however, is typically neither simple nor straightforward, because a wide range of relevant factors need to be considered. These factors—some overt and some covert—will, or at least should, impact upon the decisions that are made. In order to ensure that the process minimizes the potential for the development of the hidden curriculum, these issues *must* be openly and honestly considered. As already noted, ethical decision making depends on earnest efforts to understand and take account of the various value structures that may be in play and an openness to all opportunities to advance the welfare of those being served. These two requirements of ethical decision making alone dictate that curriculum designers must be alert to the issues that may play a role in the selection (consciously or otherwise) of alternative or additional educational objectives for deaf and hard of hearing students.

There are many issues that are relevant to the process of decision making regarding the selection or creation of curriculum objectives. For the most part, these issues relate to values and beliefs of the people most intimately involved in the curriculum development process. Among many others, these issues include:

- the particular social and cultural perspective on deafness held by the child's family, and significant others such as early intervention specialists, teachers, therapists, doctors, and ultimately, by the child;
- the particular significance given to certain educational, therapeutic, and/or medical interventions by those same individuals;
- individual teachers' ideologies and perceptions of the special learning needs of deaf and hard of hearing learners and their beliefs about what constitutes sound educational practice for students who are deaf or hard of hearing; and
- the worldview and social circumstances of the child's family, and ultimately, of the child.

The Significance of Perspective on Deafness

The issue of "perspective" on deafness is potentially a very powerful influence on the shape of the curriculum—both official and actual—and demands careful and thorough consideration. The extent to which the curriculum may need to be amended or augmented will be greatly influenced by the perspective on deafness and deaf people that is adopted by those involved in the curriculum development process. Typically, discussion of perspectives on deafness identifies two broad ways of conceptualizing deafness. Broadly defined these are a "sociocultural" perspective and a "mainstream culture" or "disability" perspective.

The sociocultural perspective recognizes deafness as essentially a socially constructed phenomenon. This is often referred to as a Deaf community perspective (capitalization intended). For members of the Deaf community "being Deaf" means membership of a social group that in many ways is characteristic of linguistic and cultural minorities. Such features include the voluntary organization of groups and networks, endogamous marital patterns, a shared historical awareness, respect for community behavioral norms, and the use of a common language (i.e., a natural sign language such as Auslan, British Sign Language, or American Sign Language) (Padden & Humphries 1988; Power 1992; Reagan, 1990). Most significantly, people who adopt a cultural perspective on deafness tend to view deafness as a social issue and not one of impairment or pathology. From this perspective there is very high value associated with bilingualism in sign language and a spoken language (i.e., in a written and possibly spoken form) as an important life outcome for people who are deaf.

The sociocultural or Deaf community perspective contrasts with the view of the mainstream or dominant culture—that is, the perspective of the hearing world. From this perspective, deafness is most commonly viewed as a condition to be either avoided or ameliorated by either (or some combination of) medical or educational/therapeutic interventions. This perspective recognizes hearing impairment as a significant potential impediment to the development and use of spoken language skills. A person with impaired hearing is not seen as a member of separate community but rather as a member of the broader "hearing" community who has a disability that is to be overcome or ameliorated. This is the view most commonly adopted by, and in relation to, people who are post-lingually deafened (i.e., people who have lost their hearing after they have acquired spoken language and have a more mainstream cultural view of the world). Regardless of the degree of impairment or the age at which it occurred, however, the identifying feature of this perspective is the belief in the preeminence of the majority community language and oral communication (i.e., speech and listening/lipreading) as the main means of communication for people who are deaf or have impaired hearing. Although, from this perspective, there is recognition of the shared experience of people with impaired hearing, there is typically no highly organized social cohesion between members of this group, as in the case of the Deaf community.

As already indicated there is broad general agreement that certain characteristics of hearing impairment suggest the need for specific curriculum objectives. Clearly then, the perspective that is adopted in regard to deafness will strongly influence individual perceptions of what those characteristics may be. Fundamentally, people who adopt one or other of the two perspectives will perceive an individual who has a hearing impairment in quite different ways. It follows therefore that curriculum decisions, such as decisions about objectives, will be influenced by the particular social construction of deafness that is adopted. To some extent, either wittingly or unwittingly, these perspectives will influence the decisions about the extent and nature of any alternative or additional curriculum objectives that may be considered necessary to address the particular learning needs of a student with impaired hearing.

For the individual who perceives the child's situation from a sociocultural perspective, there will be a range of learning outcomes that will likely be preconceived as being both necessary and desirable. Not least among these will undoubtedly be the need for the development of a sign language. Alternatively, the individual who adopts a hearing-mainstream perspective will perceive the child as a member of the broader society who has a significant disability, and therefore will see potentially very different priorities. Not least among these will most likely be a high priority on the development of spoken language skills, particularly speech skills.

How can there be room for such widely differing constructions of the same circumstance—even before individual differences have been considered? What is an ethical response to the potential for alternative perspectives to realize differential outcomes in terms of the design of curriculum objectives for deaf students? Is there a correct perspective to adopt? Is it reasonable to accept that different individual perspectives by those most closely involved in the curriculum development process could realize different objectives (and potentially different outcomes) for different students even when those students may otherwise have similar characteristics? There is a need to acknowledge such questions as important issues for consideration in curriculum development. To this end, there is a need for a process that seeks to address all such issues as part of the curriculum decision-making process.

Dealing with Prevailing Issues and Alternative Perspectives in the Curriculum Development Process

The potential clash of the two perspectives on deafness described earlier is meant to be illustrative of just one of a large range of issues and dilemmas that relate not only to decision making about relevant objectives for deaf students but also to every other decision that is made in regard to the range of curriculum questions posed earlier. Each of those issues has the potential to be the source of differential decisions in curriculum design for deaf and hard of hearing students according to the different positions on those issues that may be adopted by the players in the process.

Some curriculum decisions will be taken as a consequence of law or other administrative controls of the state—although, as we have observed in the second scenario at the commencement of this chapter, there is often considerable scope for the special educational system to opt out of such guidelines. Other decisions may be seen as coming naturally to a competent professional and would, therefore, have a considerable prospect of producing consensus in any situation. Many curriculum decisions, however, will have the potential for significant variation according to the impact of particular circumstances, issues, and perspectives on those issues. There can be no safeguard against the development of a hidden curriculum or an official/actual curriculum gap without an engagement with those issues and a considered response to the dilemmas they create. To this end, there needs to be a component of the curriculum development and implementation process that requires curriculum developers to consider all of the alternative issues and perspectives. Such a process should then allow for genuinely participatory decision making by all involved.

Being guided by the principles outlined in Figure 8.1, it is evident that approaching the task of curriculum design and implementation without having fully considered all perspectives and all of the potential issues would be clearly unethical. There can be no effective decisions made without a clear understanding of the context and potential ramifications of those decisions both in the immediate context as well as in broader and future contexts. To this end, Skilbeck (1976) suggested that the key factor in any curriculum development process was an effective strategy for analyzing the curriculum development context or "situation." He argued that there was a need for such a "situational analysis" to focus on all relevant issues and perspectives through a formal process of considering all relevant external and internal factors. Figure 8.2 provides a list of the factors that Skilbeck suggested should be systematically considered in a formal process of situational analysis.

Although they are not elaborated upon here, these factors provide a very useful guide for curriculum developers. I would argue that the complexities of curriculum development for deaf and hard of hearing learners underscore the need for such a process as a basis for ensuring that all relevant issues and perspectives are clearly identified and considered. To approach the task of curriculum design without considering the impact of all relevant issues and alternative perspectives is to do a fundamental disservice to the students whom we set out to serve. To fail to

---

External
- cultural and social changes and expectations, including parental expectations, employer requirements, community assumptions and values, changing relationships (e.g., between adults and children), and ideology;
- educational-system requirements and challenges (e.g., policy statements examinations, local authority expectations or demands or pressures, curriculum projects, educational research);
- the changing nature of the subject matter to be taught;
- the potential contribution of teacher-support systems (e.g., teacher training colleges, research institutes, etc.);
- flow of resources into the school.

Internal
- pupils: aptitudes, abilities, and defined educational needs;
- teachers: values, attitudes, skills, knowledge, experience, special strengths and weaknesses, roles;
- school ethos and political structure: common assumptions and expectations, methods of achieving conformity to norms and dealing with deviance;
- material resources, including plant, equipment, and the potential for enhancing these;
- perceived and felt problems and shortcomings in the existing curriculum.

FIGURE 8.2.   Factors that constitute the curriculum development "situation," as identified by Skilbeck (1976, pp. 142–143).

acknowledge that a particular social perspective on deafness may lead to the adoption of a set of objectives for a deaf student that are not consonant with that student's current or future social circumstances may result in a situation where both educational means and ends are subsequently questioned or rejected by that student and his or her cultural community. There are, for example, unfortunate examples of young deaf students and deaf adults who have come to question, often bitterly, the lack of inclusion of sign language and deaf culture in their educational experiences (Jacobs, 1989). Similarly, some deaf people educated in more socioculturally defined programs have come to question their lack of access to assistive technologies for hearing and their lack of programmed opportunity to develop expressive spoken language skills (Bertling, 1994). Clearly, there are issues relating to current and future cultural affiliation that must be considered in curriculum design.

The point of this discussion is not to suggest that all curriculum decisions for deaf and hard of hearing students should become so generic and "all-inclusive" as to attempt to be all things to all students by reflecting all possible alternative social perspectives on deafness in all aspects of the curriculum. Clearly, such an approach would not be logical, practical, or ethical. The point is simply that curriculum decisions must be fully informed and must be made with cognizance by all involved of the full range of potential outcomes and the full range of alternative perspectives on those potential outcomes. Alternative perspectives and alternative responses to key issues must be fairly and honestly considered. The important issue is not what the ultimate decision is but that it was made with the full ranges of issues and possibilities being patent for all concerned. Such open consideration may lead to altogether different decisions or may, at least, lead to the inclusion of additional objectives, experiences, or approaches to assessment that may not have otherwise been considered.

Such a process cannot be left to chance. Simply acknowledging the need for a process of situational analysis is not enough. Sockett (1976) warned of the danger of simply paying lip service to such a process, noting that it is possible to act too hastily in an attempt to consider the relevant issues and alternative perspectives and to miss some important aspects. Similarly, he argued that there are dangers in using a formal plan of action that is so rigid as to either (a) unnecessarily limit or exclude the treatment of some issues or perspectives that should be considered as part of the process or, (b) treat all issues equally when some should be given higher priority.

There can be no "cookbook" approach to situational analysis in curriculum development for deaf and hard of hearing students. The example issues already identified in regard to the question of setting objectives are merely illustrative of the type that should be considered. Properly administered, it is to be expected that the process of situational analysis will generate a long list of issues and perspectives that beg consideration in the decision-making process on all curriculum questions. Ethically, I would argue that there could be no substitute for such a process. Anything less provides the potential for the development of the types of hidden and other undesirable curriculum components that were evidenced in the two scenarios at the beginning of this chapter.

REVISITING THE ETHICAL DILEMMAS

As indicated at the outset, the dilemmas that confront Roslyn (Sui May's support teacher) in the first scenario, and Jenny in the second scenario, concern the need for well-informed and responsible decision making. How might the outcomes of these respective situations be served by the application of the principles that have been outlined herein? As in other parts of this chapter, there is space to respond only briefly to this question by focusing on a few example issues in each case.

In the case of Sui May, an effectively conducted situational analysis would undoubtedly provide a wealth of issues and information for consideration at both the internal and external levels. At the level of external analysis there would be a wide range of important cultural and social expectations, parental expectations, and community values to be considered. Further, there would be a need to consider the issues generated by the requirements of the educational system and the challenges that those requirements may create for Sui May. The analysis would also necessarily involve consideration of the information provided by educational research—particularly the research literature on the efficacy of the alternative educational and communication approaches that are indicated as possible alternatives for Sui May. Specifically, for example, there would be cause to consider the known limitations of the alternative approaches and how Sui May's parents might be informed about these in an accessible manner as a basis for their active participation in the decision-making process.

At the internal level of analysis, two obvious issues for consideration, among the myriad of other potential issues, would be (1) Sui May's aptitudes, abilities, and likely communication and educational needs, and (2) the values and educational priorities held by Roslyn. The examination of these issues, and the subsequent process of curriculum design, would require the application of high standards of professional behavior (i.e., as suggested in Figure 8.1). In particular, the process would demand a high level of professional competence and the need for recognition of professional limitations. There would unquestionably be a need for professional competence in the conduct of any assessment of communication skills and a need for awareness of the areas in which those professional skills may be limited. It is possible, for example, that there would be a need to enlist the additional support or assistance of the speech pathologist and/or someone with specific skills in sign language assessment. Further, ethical practice would dictate the need for transparency in effectively reporting the results of those assessments to all concerned.

In regard to the issue of identifying and clarifying the relevant values held by the players in the process, there would be a particular need for a careful and considered strategy. Clearly, it would be extremely important for Roslyn and others to be fully aware of the personal and community values held by Sui May's parents, her extended family, and the various communities (both specific and general) from which Sui May comes. However, in order for Roslyn to be effective in determining and presenting the educational options and potential benefits effectively, it would be necessary for her to be personally cognizant of her own perspectives and potential biases. This would necessitate a full articulation of her tacit and explicit assumptions, values, and perspectives on deafness as well as her own perspectives on the beliefs and aspirations that are held by Sui May's family. Cognizance and, if appropriate, disclosure, of these personal attributes would be necessary to ensure that her perception of, and response to, the issues and information identified by the situational analysis process was not unwittingly influenced. Such a processes is fundamental in guarding against the development of a hidden curriculum.

In the case of Jenny and her class, several aspects of the conduct of the situational analysis process warrant comment as examples of ethical practice. At the level of external analysis it would be important to consider relevant social expectations, parental expectations, and community values in regard to normal progression through the established age-equivalent levels of the specified core curriculum. In this regard, there would be a particular need to consider the specific educational-system requirements and the challenges that those requirements may create for the particular group of students. Any decision to deviate from those standards should be based on a careful analysis of all aspects of the children's situation with the resultant information being made explicit and available to all of the relevant stakeholders—parents, school authorities, and system authorities—as a basis for active participation in the decision-making process.

Also at the external level, the school's gradual move to adopt a sign language-based approach in preference to a total (simultaneous) communication approach should be part of a process of analysis that considers a wide range of issues. Not least among these should be consideration of all relevant research—educational and linguistic—and the perceived problems and shortcomings in the existing curriculum arrangements in regard to language and communication. From an ethical practice perspective, the important word here is "all." The process of situational analysis would require investigation of all available research. An ethical response to this imperative would dictate that the investigation should be open and exhaustive, not narrow and limited. It should consider the available evidence on the advantages of the new approach and not just the evidence on the shortcomings of the existing methods. Indeed, this has not always been the approach of our field in regard to such issues. Stewart (1992) made this same observation and noted that an open research-based approach was necessary as a basis for curriculum change in regard to language and communication issues. He noted that such an approach to curriculum change "would offer an alternative to the long-standing tendency of the field to promote one approach by denigrating the effectiveness of the other" (p. 81).

Ethically, the process of review of the research literature should consider all available studies investigating the likely efficacy of a change in communication policy and the full ramifications of such a transition in regard to both classroom practice and home-based interaction. In particular, there would be a need to consider the literature on the known and probable benefits and limitations of such a change in regard to deaf students' long-term academic achievement, majority language development, and psychosocial development. In the absence of the availability of such research, there would be a need to consider alternative means for obtaining the necessary theoretical underpinning and actual evidence to support the change.

Associated with this process of investigation would necessarily be a strategy to ensure that the children's parents were informed in an accessible manner about the available evidence on the benefits and limitations of the alternative approaches as a basis for their participation in the decision-making process. Such a process would undoubtedly be time-consuming and difficult but would be a fundamental and ethical step in such an important curriculum change process.

Among the many important issues to be considered at the internal level of analysis of Jenny's curriculum situation would be the values and educational priorities held by the school's other teachers. As in the previous case, this would mean nothing less than a full articulation of their tacit and explicit assumptions, values, and perspectives on deafness as a basis for ensuring that no relevant perspectives were either overlooked or overemphasised in curriculum design.

These few brief examples do not describe the full potential of situational analysis process to reveal important and influential issues and perspectives as part of the curriculum development process. These examples do serve, however, to demonstrate the importance of the process as a basis for ethical and effective curriculum decision making, and as an important component in a strategy to diminish the possibility of a hidden or unofficial curriculum.

CONCLUSIONS

I have endeavored to show that we are best served by a definition of curriculum that is broad and encompasses all of the arrangements that are made for deaf and hard of hearing students' learning. Such a definition clearly highlights the importance of decision making in curriculum development and implementation and, as a consequence, I have indicated the need for a set of well-informed and ethical practices to be employed in making those decisions. My emphasis has been on the need for consideration of all relevant issues and available information. Every time we make a decision in curriculum development we should be in a position to ensure that the decision is based on the best possible information, well-reasoned argument, and sound evidence, and not in mere expediency because it is the easiest, simplest, least expensive, or least confronting course of action. Ethically, we face these decisions with the imperative that our decisions should be taken with a view to providing for the greatest possible good while ensuring the least possible likelihood of harm for the students in our charge.

As curriculum developers for students with hearing impairments, we have no specific code of ethics to guide our work. I have argued, however, that there are both broad principles of ethical professional behavior and specific principles of good curriculum design that are capable of guiding our efforts toward effective and ethically sound outcomes for deaf or hard of hearing students.

REFERENCES

Bell, R., & Pitt, D. (1976). The case of Mackenzie. In R. Bell, D. Pitt, & M. Skilbeck (Eds.), *The scope of curriculum study* (pp. 7–44). Milton Keynes: The Open University Press.

Bertling, T. (1994). *A child sacrificed to the deaf culture.* Wilsonville, OR: Kodiak Media Group.

Brady, L. (1990). *Curriculum development* (3rd ed.). Sydney: Prentice-Hall.

Bunch, G. O. (1987). *The curriculum and the hearing-impaired student.* Boston: Little Brown.

Claydon, L., Knight, T., & Rado, M. (1977). *Curriculum and culture: Schooling in a pluralist society.* Sydney: George Allen & Unwin.

Education Department of Victoria. (1985). *Curriculum frameworks P-12: An introduction.* Melbourne: Author.

Jackson, P. W. (1968). *Life in classrooms.* New York: Holt, Rinehart and Winston.

Jacobs, L. M. (1989). *A deaf adult speaks out* (3rd ed.). Washington, DC: Gallaudet University Press.

Ladd, J. (1980). The quest for a code of professional ethics: An intellectual and moral confusion, In R. Chalk, M. S. Frankel, & S. B. Chafer (Eds.), *AAAS professional ethics project: Professional ethics activities in the scientific and engineering societies* (pp. 154–159). Washington, DC: American Association for the Advancement of Science.

Moores, D. F. (1990). Research in educational aspects of deafness. In D. F. Moores & K. P. Meadow-Orlans (Eds.), *Educational and developmental aspects of deafness* (pp. 11–24). Washington, DC: Gallaudet University Press.

Padden, C., & Humphries, T. (1988). *Deaf in America: Voices from a culture.* Cambridge, MA: Harvard University Press.

Power, D. (1992). Deaf people: A linguistic minority or a disability group? *Australian Disability Review,* 4–92, 43–48.

Reagan, T. (1990). Cultural considerations in the education of deaf children. In D. F. Moores & K. P. Meadow-Orlans (Eds.), *Educational and developmental aspects of deafness* (pp. 73–84). Washington, DC: Gallaudet University Press.

Seddon, T. (1983). The hidden curriculum: An overview. *Curriculum Perspectives, 3*(1), 1–6.

Skilbeck, M. (1976). Appendix 2. The curriculum-development process: A model for school use. In D. Lawton, W. Prescott, P. Gammage, J. Greenwald, & H. McMahon (Eds.), *The child, the school, and society* (pp. 141–144). Milton Keynes: The Open University Press.

Sockett, H. (1976). *Designing the curriculum.* London: Open Books.

Stewart, D. (1992). Initiating reform in total communication programs. *The Journal of Special Education, 26,* 68–84.

Tyler, R. W. (1949). *Basic principles of curriculum and instruction.* Chicago: University of Chicago Press.

APPENDIX

Important or Main Points

- We are best served by a broad rather than a narrow definition of curriculum. "The curriculum" refers to all of the arrangements that are made for students' learning.
- Curriculum development is fundamentally a process of effective and informed decision making.

- It must be recognized that the decisions involved in curriculum development and implementation are all made in a particular social context and are inherently value-laden.
- Curriculum is a wide-ranging concept that includes both official and unofficial components and outcomes. Any curriculum is likely to be based, at least in part, on a set of assumptions and behavior patterns that may not be consciously articulated but will nevertheless reflect a particular set of values or beliefs—the so-called hidden curriculum.
- There are four questions that serve to define the decisions that must be made by curriculum developers—What should be taught? How should it be taught? How should the learning experiences be ordered and organized? How are we to know when desired learning outcomes have been achieved?
- A wide range of "factors" need to be considered in addressing the four curriculum questions.
- In order to ensure that the process minimizes the potential for the development of the hidden curriculum, these factors must be openly and honestly considered in the context of a framework for ethical decision making.
- Ethical decision making depends on earnest efforts to understand and take account of the various value structures that may be in play and openness to all opportunities to advance the welfare of those being served.
- A process of "situational analysis" (Skilbeck, 1976) provides a means for curriculum developers to determine and consider all of the relevant factors as a basis for participatory decision making by all involved.
- Simply acknowledging the need for a process of situational analysis is not enough. Ethical practice demands an effectively implemented strategy for analyzing the situation—a process that considers a wide range of issues.
- Properly administered, it is to be expected that the process of situational analysis will generate a long list of issues and perspectives that beg consideration in the curriculum development process.

Follow-up References or Suggestions

The references that follow include texts and curriculum documents that focus specifically on curriculum development for deaf or hard of hearing students and/or actual curriculum documents for that population. To the extent that you may consult them, I would encourage you to ask a number of relevant questions in regard to each one.

What are the values or perspectives on deafness of the authors that are revealed in the publications? To what extent have the authors accounted for alternative perspectives on deafness and how have these alternatives been juxtaposed? Are the curriculum issues that are considered in the publication treated as variables or constants? How could the documents be used in the context of a curriculum design process that is founded in a process of situational analysis and open decision making? In the absence of such a process, what would be the consequence of unquestioningly adopting the perspectives and treatment of issues offered in these publications?

- The following are sample resources with a broad focus on curriculum for students who are deaf or hard of hearing.

1. Bunch, G. O. (1987). *The curriculum and the hearing-impaired student: Theoretical and practical considerations.* Boston: Little, Brown.
2. Johnson, R., Liddell, S., & Erting, C. (1989). *Unlocking the curriculum: Principles for achieving access in deaf education, Gallaudet Research Institute Working Papers 89–3.* Washington, DC: Gallaudet University.
3. Knight, P., & Swanick, R. (1996). *Bilingualism and the education of deaf children: Advances in practice. Conference Proceedings—June 29th 1996.* Leeds: The School of Education, University of Leeds.
4. Luetke-Stahlman, B. (1999). *Language across the curriculum: When students are deaf or hard of hearing.* Hillsboro, OR: Butte.
5. Luetke-Stahlman, B., & Luckner, J. (1991). *Effectively educating students with hearing impairments.* New York: Longman.

- The following are sample curriculum documents and resources for deaf and hard of hearing students.

1. Clark School for the Deaf—Speech Curriculum Committee. (1995). *Speech development and improvement: Curriculum series.* Northampton, MA: Clark School for the Deaf.
2. Greenberg, M., & Kusche, C. (1993). *Promoting social and emotional development in deaf children: The PATHS project.* Seattle, WA: University of Washington Press.
3. Goldberg-Strout, J., & Van Ert Windle, J. (1992). *Developmental Approach to Successful Listening II (DASL II).* Houston, TX: Houston School for Deaf Children, Resource Point.
4. KDES (Kendall Demonstration Elementary School) faculty and staff. (1989). *Preschool curriculum guide.* Washington, DC: Pre-College Programs.
5. Northcott, W. H. (Ed.). (1972). *Curriculum guide; hearing impaired children—birth to three years—and their parents.* Washington, DC: AG Bell Association for the Deaf.
6. Odom, S., Bender, M., Stein, M., Doran, L., Houden, P., McInnes, M, Gilbert, M., Deklyen, M., Speltz, M., & Jenkins, J. (1988). *The integrated preschool curriculum, procedures for socially integrating young handicapped and normally developing children.* Seattle, WA: University of Washington Press.

Ethical Questions for Consideration

- Given the inevitability of alternative "perspectives" on deafness is it possible for individual teachers of deaf and hard of hearing students to ethically "manage" the curriculum development process and ensure against an active hidden curriculum?

- Considering your answer to the previous question, is there an alternative to teacher coordination of the curriculum development process?
- Given the impact of new technologies, is it likely that the question of specialized or alternate curricula for deaf students will cease to be an issue?
- What is the role of the deaf student as a participant in the curriculum development process? For students who are too young to accept that role is there a role for someone other than their parents as an advocate for their perspective? If so, under what circumstances would this alternative advocacy be appropriate?
- Given the model for curriculum decision making that has been outlined in this chapter, how can the specialist skills and firmly held views (perspectives) on deafness of some teachers be accommodated in the context of such an approach? Is teacher specialization a problem in this context? If so, are such characteristics problematic in all curriculum contexts or only in some (e.g., early intervention as opposed to school level)?
- Given the ideas outlined in this chapter, is there a role for commercially produced curricula documents for deaf or hard of hearing students?
- Given the imperative to pursue core curriculum objectives that exist in many countries, is it realistic to seek to deliver such regular curriculum outcomes for deaf or hard of hearing students in the regular time frame? Why? Why not?
- Whose interests, if any, are served by hidden curriculum in the context of education for deaf or hard of hearing students? Is it possible to reveal and incorporate a hidden curriculum into an official curriculum?
- Do elements of the hidden curriculum assume greater importance in formal or informal learning situations? If so, what are the implications for teachers?
- To what extent, if any, can a teacher minimize a hidden curriculum? Is it possible for teaching to be a completely intentional and cooperative activity?
- Stewart (1992) noted the importance of educational research as a basis for curriculum change in regard to communication approaches for students who are deaf. Specifically, he suggested that a research-based strategy "…would offer an alternative to the longstanding tendency of the field to promote one approach by denigrating the effectiveness of the other" (p. 81). What should be the role of educational research in the curriculum decision-making process—particularly the curriculum change process? Is there a role for situation-specific (applied) research as a necessary part of that process?

9

ETHICS AND THE PREPARATION OF TEACHERS OF THE DEAF

DAVID A. STEWART

AUTHOR INTRODUCTION

I began my career teaching at the Jericho Hill School for the Deaf in Vancouver, Canada, during the last of those tranquil days of the 1970s, when there were little or no hostilities in the field about signing. Sign language users and English signers sat at the same table and talked, not about how they signed but how they taught. Then came the 1980s and I took up a position at Southern University and then Michigan State University to prepare teachers of the deaf. What I then encountered was in sharp contrast to my days teaching middle school and high school deaf students. Everyone had suddenly become an expert about signing— their way of signing. There was no other way. Scholarly discussions about teaching deaf children always ended up being a battle about how a teacher should communicate. My own students at the university were choosing sides despite my best efforts to try and convince them that our moral obligations as teachers lie in doing what is right for a deaf child.

Today, I sense a cleansing wind blowing through the field. Teachers are once again looking at what they are doing in the classroom in the area of instruction. They have come to realize that there never will be a time when a single teaching methodology or communication philosophy will satisfy the educational needs of all of their students. They are leaving their posts as sentinels for a particular philosophical belief and looking instead at who it is that they are teaching this year and what it is that each of these deaf children really need from the teacher. In short, they are becoming ethically responsible for the education of their students.

A CASE TO CONSIDER

Let's say you are a righteous person. You are the type of person to do what you believe is morally responsible. When you became a teacher of the deaf, you knew that you would always do what you thought was in the best interest of your deaf students. You are aware of the many controversies that exist in the field of deaf education, but thus far, your commitment to ethics has kept you satisfied with all of the decisions you have made. You work in a school for the deaf and one day in June you make a rather bold statement at an individualized education plan (IEP) meeting, when you suggest that Joan, an eleventh grader, would be better off returning to her home school district for the remaining two years of her education. You based your decision on the fact that Joan is far ahead all of her classmates in all subject matters, your present school does not have a challenging science and mathematics program for her, and she has expressed a strong interest to attend a state university upon graduation. Because Joan attended a school for the deaf throughout her school years, you felt that if she spent two years in a high school with hearing peers and studying in a strong academic program, that would help her when she went to a university. The parents agree with you and the IEP is completed. In August, just before school is to begin you learn that a teacher at your school who is also your best friend has been laid off because of declining enrollment. You feel sorry for your friend because you know that her husband had just lost his job, and they have three children to support. A week later, you find out that Joan's IEP team is being reconvened because of a technical error that was made on the IEP which was completed in June. Just before the meeting, your principal informs you that if Joan stays at the school for the deaf, the teacher who was laid off will be called back to work. Moreover, the principal is going to reopen the discussion about transferring Joan back to her home school district because she feels that Joan is a good role model at the school for the deaf and it would be a shame to lose her. Would you change your mind at the IEP meeting and recommend that Joan remain at the school for the deaf?

INTRODUCTION

What would Socrates do? If Socrates was a teacher of the deaf today his colleagues at the school for the deaf would have soundly chastised him for being a traitor at the IEP meeting described. Who would recommend that a top student be sent to a different school? After all, educating deaf students is, in part, a numbers game in that the more students a program has the more resources and program options that are available. Deaf students who are high achievers academically are great recruitment tools for their school programs. When Socrates agreed to work in a school for the deaf, he had come into a school culture characterized by the mind-set that schools for the deaf are the best environment for educating most deaf children. He quickly learned that a happy symbiosis seldom existed between schools for the deaf and mainstreamed programs for deaf students in public school systems.

To address this situation, Socrates would have to remove himself from the politics of the field and the emotions that he might have stemming from his friend losing her job because of a decision he had made. In fact, removing oneself from the emotional context of a situation is one of the first steps toward managing the ethical issues embedded in the situation. Socrates, being a philosopher, would turn to a set of principles that would help guide him toward making the right decision. Frankema (1973) summarized the principles that Socrates uses to help him bring ethical issues into focus:

> Socrates first lays down some points about the approach to be taken. To begin with, we must not let our decision be determined by our emotions, but must examine the question and follow the best reasoning. We must try to get our facts straight and to keep our minds clear. Questions like this can and should be settled by reason. (p. 2)

And then Frankema continued:

> Secondly, we cannot answer such questions by appealing to what people generally think. They may be wrong. We must try to find an answer we ourselves can regard as correct. We must think for ourselves. Finally, we ought never to do what is morally wrong. The only question we need to answer is whether what is proposed is right or wrong, not what will happen to us, what people will think of us, or how we feel about what has happened. (p. 2)

It is of interest to note that one of Socrates' teaching techniques was to pursue excellence in his students by continuously asking them questions to help them think through situations. When dealing with questions of ethics, each person must objectively pursue what he or she thinks is the correct thing to do. In essence, this is what ethics education is all about—teaching people to think about situations and bring their own sense of ethics to bear on the decisions that are made.

FROM THE BEGINNING

When people decide to become teachers, they are making a moral commitment to themselves, students, parents, and society to provide school children with an education that will make them productive citizens in the community. Ideally, this commitment aims to help students achieve their academic and vocational potential. This moral commitment, however, is multifaceted and carries with it more than just a resolution by someone to teach well. Bull (1983) identified two moral dimensions related to teaching: political and interpersonal. He described them as follows:

> The political perspective notes that public education involves the exercise of governmental power over citizens and observes that any such exercise, including that in which teachers engage, must meet appropriate moral standards. The second, the interpersonal perspective, notes that teachers and students are involved in a particular kind of personal relationship that imposes moral responsibilities upon its participants. (p. 70)

At the political level, education is guided by formal decisions made by the legislature, members of a state board of education, local school boards, and other school governing bodies. In special education, federal laws in the United States such as the Individuals with Disabilities Education Act (IDEA) are a display of federal power affecting the manner in which local school districts educate children with disabilities. Knowledge of these laws and recognizing the power of state and local governments in education are important ingredients in the preservice curriculum for teachers of the deaf. But future teachers need to know more than just the nature and specifics of these laws. They also need to explore the moral obligations of society that brought about the enactment, for example, of IDEA's predecessor, the Education of All Handicapped Children's Act in 1975. The outcomes of IDEA should also be explored by examining such issues as how might the education of deaf children be different today in the absence of such federal laws. Or examining the moral dilemma that school boards face when the cost of educating children with disabilities is viewed by the public as diminishing the amount of money that is left for general education.

The moral dimension of politics in education also reveals itself informally and is especially apparent in issues relating to communication. The Milan Resolution of 1880 declared that:

> (1) given the incontestable superiority of speech over signs in restoring deaf mutes to society and in giving them an improved knowledge of language, the oral method ought to be preferred to signs; and (2) considering that the simultaneous use of speech and signs has the disadvantage of hindering speech, lip reading, and grasping of ideas, the pure oral method ought to be preferred (Moores, 2001, p. 81).

The resolution made it clear that all deaf children must learn to speak in order to be a valued member of society. This had a profound effect on the landscape of deaf education as schools for the deaf switched from signed instructions to the sole use of speech and audition for all instructional purposes. The movement to oral education placed a premium on the hiring of hearing teachers who would be able to implement the tenets of an oral education program. Of particular interest is the fact that the resolution had no legal mandate to support it. It was simply a resolution passed by a group of educators (most of whom were from Europe with only a handful of Americans) at an international convention attended by teachers and administrators of deaf children. Moreover, deaf participants were forbidden to express themselves at this conference. Nevertheless, the Milan resolution is great fodder for discussion about the ethics of stereotyping the educational needs of all deaf children.

Preservice teachers become indignant when they hear that deaf students were denied the option of being educated through the use of sign language. But do teachers have a moral obligation to espouse the use of sign language or of speech as an option in the education of deaf children? Let us explore possible answers to this question by going back to the Milan resolution to see why a resolution with no legal support could be so persuasive as a document on how to teach deaf children. Knowing the facts and being objective in making one's decision are conditions for making ethically correct decisions. At the time of the Milan resolution, there was no research to support any type of teaching methodology for educating deaf students. The best evidence of success was the achievement level of the deaf students in a program. In the nineteenth century, educators were the reporters of their student's success and hence of their program's success, real or imagined. Thus, if a group of educators of the deaf from around the world declared that a particular communication was to be the sole method of communication, would not educators elsewhere have a moral obligation to do what was best for their deaf students and therefore accept the resolution?

Such a line of reasoning is at the heart of many discussions about ethics relating to opinions about teaching deaf children that lack legal mandates. Today, there is no single method of education or communication that dominates the field. Rather, a plurality of methods have settled into the field, thus giving preservice teachers a choice of which method they would like to pursue on their way to becoming a teacher of the deaf.

The second moral dimension of teaching is associated with the interpersonal relationship between the teacher and students. Bull (1983) offered a summary of this relationship.

> From the perspective of the student, the relationship is compulsory; it is a given in their lives, and there is very little they can do to escape it. The relationship is intimate, for teachers become privy to a detailed knowledge of the character, talents, failures, dreams, and fears of their students. It is also asymmetrical because teachers' knowledge of, and responsibility for, their students is not reciprocated by students. (p. 72)

Bull's summary also considered the future.

> Finally, the relationship is pervasive in the students' present and, to some extent, future lives; teachers have a comprehensive and sustained influence on the actions, beliefs, aspirations, and motivations of their students ... students are particularly vulnerable to their teachers' actions and motivations and, therefore, that teachers have special moral responsibilities toward their students. (p. 72)

To this description we can add the interpersonal relationship between the teacher and parents. Given the research that consistently shows the importance of parents in the education of their children, it is imperative that preservice teachers understand their role in a teacher–parent relationship.

What does having a moral responsibility toward students and their parents imply for teachers of the deaf? More specifically, how can we frame moral responsibility in real terms? I am not professing to hold the answer to these questions. I am, however, offering four examples of responsibilities that can be used to stimulate debate among future teachers about ethics and teaching responsibilities:

1. Students are not the property of teachers. Therefore, teachers must respect the right of students and their parents to make decisions relating to education.
2. Teachers are to treat their deaf students fairly and ensure that the specifications of the IEP are followed.

3. A deaf child's educational needs take priority over a teacher's job security. This belief can be associated with at least two moral responsibilities for teachers. Both of these responsibilities involve the possibility of the teacher losing a student and consequently his or her job in the event that the number of students in the classroom drops below a certain critical point:

- Teachers are obligated to inform parents when they suspect that the communication methodology they use in their classrooms is not appropriate for a deaf child.
- Teachers are obligated to inform parents when they suspect that the educational placement of a deaf child in their classroom is inappropriate.

4. Teachers are purveyors of professional knowledge. They are responsible for providing parents and others with an objective interpretation of the literature relating to issues in the field. For example, a teacher might speak only of the benefits of using ASL for instructional purposes, of providing young deaf children with cochlear implants, or of the language modeling advantages of using an English sign system. This teacher may be performing a moral injustice by either intentionally withholding information about the possible downside in each of these cases or by being ignorant about the benefits of alternative options.

The benefits of preservice teachers discussing the merits of these moral responsibilities are invaluable. These discussions help them think about ethical issues as well as help prepare them for situations that might be encountered once they become teachers. Some of the questions that my students have raised include: Are teachers obligated to give parents their home phone numbers? If a phone number is given do they have to answer the phone after 11:00 P.M.? Do parents have a right to visit their child's classroom at any time with or without advance notice? If a parent is hampering a teacher's effort to teach, should the teacher or the principal address this matter to the parent? This last question is illustrated in the following actual case:

> The parents of an 8-year old deaf boy, attending a school for the deaf, objected to a teacher's use of a particular language program. After discussing the matter with the teacher and being informed that this particular program has always been used successfully in the school, the parents still demanded that the program not be used with their son. The teacher informed them that she would continue to use the program because it is a critical part of the elementary school language program. The parents then instructed their son to put his head facedown on the desk whenever the teacher began using this language program.

This case brings up the question about the moral responsibilities of parents who place the education of their children in the hands of a school. Arranging for parents of deaf children to discuss their expectations and beliefs relating to the education of their deaf children with preservice teachers can prove to be an enlightening event for all involved.

THE ETHICS OF WHAT WE TEACH TEACHERS

What is it about the ethics of teaching deaf students that preservice teachers of the deaf should be learning? Ethics is a branch of philosophy that deals with what is good and what is bad; what decisions can be said to be right and which ones are wrong; and what are people's moral obligations in their various walks of life. Behaving in an ethical manner is an important value in all societies because a path of righteousness garners trust in people. Trust is the most basic of all human behaviors required for people to live together in an orderly and systematic manner. Teachers of the deaf have been entrusted to do what is right when they teach deaf children in their own classrooms. If they are itinerant teachers, then they are trusted to provide other teachers with correct information about teaching techniques to use with deaf students. All teachers are trusted to provide parents with an objective and balanced perspective about various issues relating to the education of deaf children.

This leads to the question about what is the right thing to do in the education of deaf children. There is no simple answer to this question. All fields of education have differences of opinion when it comes to deciding how best to teach children. These differences can be political as when a state endorses English immersion for all students for whom English is a second language. Differences might also be related to interpretation as when different conclusions are drawn from the same research base and ultimately leading to contrasting teaching methodologies. Disagreement about educational outcomes will lead to the formulation of alternate curricula. These differences are, perhaps, to be expected because certainty in teaching practices is seldom a sure thing in our field. For example, no one seems to know for certain what is the best way to teach reading and writing skills despite a century of teaching and millions of dollars spent on research.

In the education of deaf children, it is a complex task to address the specific educational challenges that deafness poses. This task is often defined in terms that pit one effort against another, which creates a dichotomy in the services that are provided to deaf students. Examples of some of these dichotomies can be found in each of the following areas:

- *Communication.* A deaf student can enroll in a program that endorses the use of signed communication, an oral education program, or one that supports both.
- *Signed communication.* A program might use a form of English signing or a natural sign language like American Sign Language as the primary means of in-the-air communication.
- *Educational placement.* A deaf student can attend a school for the deaf or be placed in one of several public school programs including a self-contained classroom, and full integration with support services in a general education classroom.
- *Support services.* A mainstreamed student can have the services of an interpreter or a real-time reporter, but seldom if ever, both.

- *Auditory support.* A deaf student can receive a cochlear implant or use conventional hearing amplification systems such as hearing aids and auditory trainers.
- *Social/Culture.* The curriculum can be guided entirely by principles established for a hearing and speaking society or it can incorporate information and guidance from the cultural experiences of Deaf people.
- *Instruction.* There are numerous options in this area but one that concerns many teachers of the deaf is how best to teach English. One type of program asserts that reading and writing is the best and possibly only way to promote proficiency in English, whereas other programs assert that exposure to English in all of its modalities (e.g., speech, audition, signs, and print) is critical to the acquisition of English skills.

In each of these foregoing areas, the options presented have been around for a long time and are responses to the challenge of teaching deaf children. Yet, evaluation of their positive impact on the education of deaf children is inconclusive. This lack of research support complicates the task of establishing a responsible curriculum for the education of preservice teachers of the deaf.

Further complications arise from the fact that deaf children represent a heterogeneous population. These children bring into the classroom a host of individual characteristics, each of which may impact on their education in ways ranging from the manner in which they are taught to the location and nature of the program in which they are taught. The field is well versed in these characteristics, which include age at onset of deafness, etiology, degree of hearing loss, linguistic proficiency, ethnic background, socioeconomic status of the family, hearing status of parents, and the presence of additional disabilities (Marschark, 1997; Moores, 2001). To this list we can add the level of effective communication experienced in the home environment and the degree of authentic experiences that the child has had outside of the classroom, both of which are factors from the home environment that Stewart and Kluwin (2001) have identified as being critical to the way in which teachers design instruction.

Thus, given the diversity of deaf students it may be an unreasonable and pointless task to evaluate teaching methodologies, placement options, communication choices, and other factors in terms of what works best for the field of deaf education as a whole. For preservice teachers, then, a key question might not be what educational practice is good for "deaf children" but rather what parameters define educational practices that are effective for some groups of deaf students? If we take this one step further, and define effective educational practices as they relate to a single deaf child, then we have arrived at the ultimate level of being morally responsible for the education of that child.

ETHICS EDUCATION

No teacher wants to think that what he or she is doing is morally wrong. But if teachers are not taught about ethics as part of their preservice education, they may make decisions relating to teaching that are ethically incorrect. Thus, ethics education should be an integral part of all preparation programs for teachers of the deaf. Infusing case studies about ethical dilemmas throughout the coursework of a program is how I approach the teaching of ethics in my program.

In this section, I present a number of ethically challenging cases that require the teacher to make a decision. Making a decision is a complex process that bears interest in many areas of deaf education. For example, Case #1 touches on issues involved with support services, educational placement, job security, and instruction. Readers might identify other issues depending on the perspective they use to reflect upon the case.

In presenting these cases I do not stake out an ethical position. Nor do I attempt to delineate positions that the field of deaf education might agree upon. Ethics education and, more generally, the preparation of teachers of the deaf should not be dogmatic in informing preservice teachers about options in the field relating to instruction, placement, communication, and other matters. Options in each of these areas are available because each of them is suitable for some deaf students.

The purpose of ethics education is to provide preservice teachers with insights into situations that may require them to make moral judgments. In discussions about ethics these teachers gain practice in using their intellectual tools and hopefully acquire a commitment to ethics that will help them reflect on the decisions they will face when they become teachers. There are consequences to every decision that teachers make and purposeful deliberations about ethics will help preservice teachers anticipate these consequences. Moreover, the ethical situations that they talk about should be real and touch upon issues that require them to reexamine their own beliefs as well as to consider the arguments offered by others whose beliefs might impact on the decisions they are making.

Finally, all preservice teachers want to learn about what they should do in all of the teaching situations they will encounter once they become teachers. Being certain is a great confidence booster that can mean the difference between a good and a mediocre teacher. Unfortunately, we do not have all of the answers required to give preservice teachers the requisite knowledge and skills that they desire and need. Nevertheless, given the short time frame that most teacher preparation programs have this will mean that what they teach will to some extent be eclectic. Just as teachers must make choices about what and how they teach, so too must teacher educators. In sum, all professionals must "be responsible for consciously reflecting on the ethical reasoning capabilities and character virtues that are consistent with principled reasoning" (Schrader, 1983, p. 97).

CASE STUDIES

The Ethics of What Teacher Preparation Programs Teach

I have rarely been involved in a debate about the content of a program that prepares teachers of the deaf. What I do in my program is generally up to me.

Although I follow state guidelines with respect to much of the content, the emphasis of my program—my recruitment mantra—is something that I decide. I emphasize the use of signed communication but I also stress that teachers of the deaf must be prepared to teach under a range of communication options if they wish to satisfactorily meet the educational needs of their deaf students. Hence, in addition to sign communication, my program includes grounding in theory and practices of speech communication.

Yet, by emphasizing one type of communication over another, am I knowingly not preparing my preservice teachers for the range of students they will teach? Although there is insufficient time in teacher preparation programs to teach everything teachers need to know, as teacher educators do we have a moral obligation to inform our students about the benefits of alternative teaching strategies and communication methodologies that we might not emphasize in our own teacher preparation program? Consider the following story:

Example of Erin

Erin was a 20-year-old student thinking about what she would like to do as a teacher. She knew she wanted to teach deaf children and observed elementary total communication and oral education programs. After these visits, she decided that she liked the idea of signing to deaf students and felt that perhaps this would be her strong suit as a teacher. She also valued the role of speech in the education of deaf students and wanted to be prepared to teach and use speech in her classroom. She made an appointment with the director of a deaf education program at a university to inquire about the nature of his program. He told her that his program focuses only on oral education methods. Because Erin was already attending this university she was not wholly turned off by what she had just heard. Furthermore, she believed that speech communication was the best option for some deaf children and especially for hard of hearing children. She thought about the situation, then asked the director if she would be allowed at least some experiences with signing deaf students to compliment her training in oral education in his program. She offered to be responsible for learning to sign and was willing to stay another semester at the university in order to get supervised experiences in a signing classroom environment. At this point, the director was taken aback and became defensive about his program's course offerings. He stated that all deaf children should learn to speak and be integrated into the hearing world. With speech, he went on, a deaf child would have no need to ever learn to sign. Furthermore, deaf children who learn to sign do not acquire good speech; therefore, he would not take on a student in his teacher-training program if that student already knew how to sign or expressed any interest in learning to sign. Erin decided to apply to a different deaf education teaching training program.

Did the program director do the right thing when he told Erin that his program would not have anything to do with signing? By being honest about what his program offered, he ensured that Erin had the information necessary to make a decision about whether or not to apply to his program. Upon digesting what the director said about his approach to the preparation of teachers of the deaf, Erin was then able to make an informed decision when she chose a different program.

Let us now reexamine Erin's case from the perspective of doing what is right when preparing preservice teachers for a career in the education of deaf children. An all-important question that immediately comes to mind is whether it is ethically correct to prepare teachers of the deaf for one type of teaching (e.g., using signed communication, oral education, bilingual-bicultural education). Discussing the many possible responses to this question helps future teachers think about their own career in the field and usually makes them more open-minded to the various communication approaches that are available.

I encourage students to think not only about where they want to work upon graduation, but also where they might be working in 10 years. I highlight this discussion activity with real examples of teachers trained in a program that emphasizes signing who land jobs working in an oral program. Similarly, I have them think about the ethics of those teachers who agree to teach in a Total Communication program even though they obviously lack proficient signing skills. Both of these situations are all too common. Ultimately, it is the deaf student who suffers at the hands of teachers inadequately prepared to teach them.

The Ethics of Hanging on to One's Job

What is the ultimate responsibility of a teacher of the deaf? Many might respond that the primary goal of all teachers is to serve the needs of the field by doing what is right for the greatest number of deaf students. On the surface, this appears to be a rather obvious response to the question. But let us apply this thinking to the following case.

Example of Karen and Dan

Let's suppose that one day you spend a morning with Karen, an itinerant teacher. Karen's entire caseload consists of just five students and includes Dan, an 11-year-old boy in the fifth grade who has a severe-profound hearing loss. You observe Karen working with Dan whom she pulls out of the classroom three times a week to go over language arts activities. Dan comes from an English-speaking family but is in a French immersion school where French is spoken for all subject matter teaching, although the school's language arts classes consisted of learning English through English instructions. Dan has an eleventh-grade reading level and had consistently earned A's and B's in all of his subject matter. During these pull-out sessions, Karen usually reviews vocabu-

lary and asks comprehension questions relating to a passage that Dan is required to read aloud. When you get back to the car to drive to the next school, you ask Karen why she is spending time with Dan who obviously does not need instructional support and why she focused her lesson on reading when Dan's reading level was six grades ahead of his grade level. Her response is that Dan in fact does not need itinerant support services because he is ahead of most of the students in his class. If, however, she gave him up then she would be out of a job.

When presented with this scenario, my preservice students tend to react in disgust at Karen's behavior. This is somewhat understandable when you consider that the average age of the students is 22 years, 95% of them are unmarried and unattached, and the married ones seldom have children. Being young and idealistic, my students are therefore indignant that Karen would be concerned about her own welfare over that of her deaf students. They argue that any student with a severe hearing loss and who is doing so well in a French immersion school should be fully mainstreamed without any form of pull out. The pull-out sessions are considered detrimental to Dan's overall educational and social development because they show his hearing classmates that he is different from them.

In considering the ethics of this case, the students emphasize the importance of social conformity. They preach that teachers must do what is right for their deaf students and put their own personal needs aside. Their argument is based on Dan's academic performance and his consequential lack of need for pull-out support services.

But once these future teachers have expressed this visceral feeling I introduce the next part of the ethical dilemma.

Example of Karen and Dan Continued

The school district requires that there be at least five deaf students with IEPs requesting the services of an itinerant teacher before they can hire a teacher of the deaf to provide these services. Any number lower than five, the teacher of the deaf is then released from her teaching responsibility and the deaf students are placed on the caseload of another special education teacher who is not certified to teach deaf students.

At this point, an interesting transformation in my students' thinking begins to occur. Left to digest their own righteousness, they then begin to think about what happens to the four remaining students who will lose the support of their itinerant teacher when the teacher's caseload drops to four students.

The second passage helps the students to see the big picture. They move from panning a teacher of the deaf for being selfish about her own welfare to becoming self-righteous about the experiences and professional expertise that teachers of the deaf have. How dare any school board think that a teacher other than a teacher of the deaf can adequately meet the educational needs of deaf students when support services outside of the general education class are needed? When asked to elaborate on this expertise, the students touch upon a slate of deafness-related knowledge including language development, and the relationship between communication system(s) used and the acquisition of language. They also list audiological terminology and the classroom use of assistive listening devices, the influence of deafness on socialization skills and social maturity, use of educational interpreters, and other information that is critical in the preparation of teachers of the deaf.

In the past, most of my students have been content when they have reached this stage in their intellectualization of the scenario I have presented to them. In recent years, however, the politics of schools being responsible has affected how teachers and the community are viewing the role of schools in society. It is no longer sufficient for schools to be accountable for the academic performance of their students; they must also demonstrate some level of fiscal responsibility. This is illustrated in townships that ask their citizens to vote for funds needed to improve school facilities and programs. Many school districts cannot simply decide that the importance of teaching art, for example, justifies the expenditure of funds to build new art rooms in all of their elementary schools. The decision to spend money now rests with the voters. Thus, it is not surprising that in recent years my students have begun to include in their equation of being ethically responsible the notion of making a decision based on the common good of an entire community.

In this second example, we have seen preservice teachers shift their thinking about the educational and social welfare of a single deaf student to a broader realization about what is good for all of the students being served by a teacher of the deaf; in other words, the common good of the field of educating deaf students, to an even broader conceptualization of ethics that incorporates the common good of society. They have in effect, shifted their thinking from looking at the initial impact of making a decision on just one student's educational welfare to examining the possible long-term impact of the decision on a wider group of students, which extends beyond the sphere of special education to include all students in a school program.

During the course of this discussion, I do not push my students to arrive at some agreed-upon response to the itinerant teacher's insistence on continuing to give support services to a deaf student who was excelling academically. My goal is to provide them with opportunities for their thinking about ethics to evolve as they weave new information into their experience.

A good follow-up to the preceding example is the one in the next section. In this situation personnel of a deaf education program with declining enrollment wants to retain a deaf student despite the parent's request for placement in another program. The case touches upon a teacher's job security as well as issues about educational placement, satisfactory students progress, communication methodology, social-cultural environments, and parent choice.

Example of Main Elementary School

For many years since the passage of the Education of All Handicapped Children's Act in 1975, this school served as a center Total Com-

munication program with deaf students from surrounding areas being bussed in to take advantage of a full range of support services. At its peak, the school had 23 students and 4 teachers of the deaf. Then in the late 1980s the State Department of Education endorsed the inclusive education movement, which encouraged the education of all students with disabilities in local school districts. Main Elementary School saw the number of its deaf students drop to eight students and two teachers of the deaf. The state has a requirement that no teacher of the deaf can have more than seven students in a class. This year, a parent has requested that her 12-year-old deaf son be sent to the State School for the Deaf because she is dissatisfied with his educational progress—he reads at a second-grade level. The mother stressed that she felt it was time that the student learned to sign ASL well and that he be exposed to more deaf students his age as well as adult Deaf role models. If the student does transfer, then one of the two teachers of the deaf will be laid off. The school district's special education office and the teachers argue that the student's educational interest is best served at Main Elementary, despite a general agreement with the parent's assessment of the student's educational progress. They claim that the deaf student is an average student academically when compared to same-age deaf peers. The parent says that this rationale for retaining the student is not good enough. Although they do not voice this concern to the parent, the teachers are worried that if the school has only one teacher of the deaf, it will be less able to serve the educational needs of all the remaining deaf students.

One value of this ethical dilemma is that it helps preservice teachers realize that even during a time when the population of a state might be increasing, their job security is affected by the politics of special education, which in turn is very much at the mercy of the politics of numbers.

The Ethics of Professional Knowledge

What are a teacher's moral obligations when talking to parents, educators, and administrators outside the field of deaf education, and even preservice teachers who might be doing an internship in their classrooms? Throughout this book, the reader is reminded about the polarization of opinions that exists in matters relating to the education of deaf children. Educators and administrators often pepper their discussions with bold statements that appeal to our moral obligation to do things right:

- "If you sign to deaf children they will not learn to speak well."
- "If deaf children learn to sign, they will become careless with their speech."
- "Every deaf child has a right to learn ASL as their first language."
- "This is a hearing world, therefore every deaf child must learn to speak."

- "Deaf children will eventually become members of the Deaf community, therefore teach them to sign."
- "Don't give deaf children hearing aids because you are trying to make them hearing, which is something they will never be."
- "Giving a child a cochlear implant is denying their deafness."
- "Don't teach deaf children phonetics because they can't hear."
- "Don't send a deaf child to a mainstreamed school because he will grow up isolated and develop poor social skills."
- "Deaf children who go to a school for the deaf learn to live in a Deaf ghetto and never learn how to interact in a hearing world."

These statements are judgments of moral obligation. It is someone telling you (e.g., a teacher, an administrator, a parent, a medical practitioner) in a frank manner how you ought to be thinking about something or, more to the point, what you should be doing. There is little evidence in any of these statements that the speaker has even a slight doubt about what she or he believes. There is also no factual evidence supporting the finality of these statements. Even if we grant the speaker that some of these statements might hold true for a small fraction of deaf children, their dogmatic tone leaves little room for discussion of alternative perspectives and consequently for discussion of what exactly teachers should know about how best to teach deaf children.

What, then, is the place of judgments of moral obligations in the preparation of future teachers of the deaf? Obviously, there are many that are indisputable such as those relating to safety—all teachers must protect the safety of their students and teachers must not physically or emotionally harm their students. Equality—teachers must not discriminate against students on the basis of gender or race; and certainly, fairness—teachers will treat all students fairly including in the manner in which they award grades.

But what about moral obligations such as the ones stated previously? Must teachers take a moral stand when it comes to matters relating to communication and language, educational placement, and social-cultural issues relating to the Deaf community and society at large? Given the lack of research support, it might appear to be a risky venture for any teacher to take an unqualified stand on any of these matters. Moreover, long before we approach the question of doing what is right in how we teach deaf children, the question of what is normal and appropriate for deaf children must be addressed. For example, are hearing teachers obligated to view the culture of their hearing and speaking society as a benchmark? If hearing and speaking is the norm, do teachers of the deaf need to seek educational solutions that will help normalize deaf students so that they are more like their hearing peers? If most of society feels that deaf children should learn to speak and rely on amplification, can teachers be impartial to this sentiment? Is the desire of the majority in society the key to the way we communicate with deaf children? If the answer to any of these questions is yes, are we not then being ethically irresponsible in our disregard for the values of the Deaf community—a community that is the product of our educational system?

CONCLUSIONS

Teacher educators are teachers too. What they teach and how they teach it tells us a lot about their philosophies of teaching. This is why we have differences in how programs approach the preparation of future teachers despite all programs usually falling under a common set of state standards. These differences do result, in part, from the limited amount of time that teacher educators are allowed to teach. The time constraint forces programs to be selective in the nature and extent of the content they choose to teach. Nevertheless, preservice teachers have a right to a comprehensive and balanced perspective of the field. To meet this moral obligation teacher educators must make careful and objective decisions about the materials they use in their classrooms and the ideas they espouse. This includes their selection of readings for their courses, the school sites they choose to visit, and the guest speakers they invite to their classes. Thus, the professional knowledge that teacher educators impart to their students is a reflection of their own ethical standards.

Ethics is about being fair. Teachers are vested with much power, and fairness can take on many shades of meaning. The same thing can be said about teacher educators. Ethics education is not just about teaching preservice teachers about what is right and what is wrong. Ethics education is about preparing teachers to consider the facts of a situation, think for themselves when making a decision, and ensure that their decision is not morally wrong. If we follow the spirit of the IEP, then we must ensure that the cadre of teachers in the field are well prepared to recognize differences in the educational needs of their deaf students and to make decisions that are in each child's best interest.

Knowledge alone is only one part of an ethics education program. Preservice teachers will benefit from discussion about ethics that is infused throughout their teacher preparation program. Case studies and examples can be used to present students with situations that encourage them to think about the morality inherent in various situations. Discussion about a case helps them "see what is at stake in a case and to develop their capacity for ethical reflection" (Strike, 1983, p. 114). We want all teachers to be able to listen to the facts of a situation, think clearly about these facts and the possible responses to the situation, then make an objective decision about what action to take. This is what Socrates would do.

REFERENCES

Bull, B. L. (1983). Ethics in the preservice curriculum. In K. A. Strike & P. L. Ternasky (Eds.), *Ethics for professionals in education: Perspectives for preparation and practice* (pp. 69–83). New York: Teachers College.

Frankena, W. (1973). *Ethics*. Englewood Cliffs, NJ: Prentice-Hall.

Marschark, M. (1997). *Raising and educating a deaf child*. New York: Oxford University Press.

Moores, D. F. (2001). *Educating the deaf: Psychology, principles, and practices* (5th ed.). Boston: Houghton Mifflin.

Schrader, D. E. (1983). Lawrence Kohlberg's approach and the moral education of education professionals. In K. A. Strike & P. L. Ternasky (Eds.), *Ethics for professionals in education: Perspectives for preparation and practice* (pp. 84–101). New York: Teachers College.

Stewart, D. A., & Kluwin, T. N. (2001). *Teaching deaf children: Content, strategies, and curriculum*. Boston: Allyn & Bacon.

Strike, K. A. (1983). Teaching ethical reasoning using cases. In K. A. Strike & P. L. Ternasky (Eds.), *Ethics for professionals in education: Perspectives for preparation and practice* (pp. 102–116). New York: Teachers College.

APPENDIX

Important or Main Points

- Teachers-in-training as well as those already practicing need to know the key elements for making ethical decisions. They must try to (a) avoid decisions being determined by emotions, (b) examine the question and follow the best reasoning, (c) get the facts straight, and (d) keep an open mind.

- Making ethical decisions involves thinking for ourselves—finding answers we regard as correct. Appealing to others to answer ethical questions is not adequate—they may be unaware of the facts, biased, or naive.

- An ethical question answered in a morally wrong way is never acceptable. Ethical decision making should not involve someone thinking What will happen to me/us? What people will think of me/us? How do I/we feel about what has happened?

- Bull (1983) identified two moral dimensions related to teaching: political and interpersonal. Both dimensions impact on ethical decision making. The political perspective involves government's adoption of appropriate moral standards for teachers. The interpersonal perspective concerns the moral responsibilities imposed on teachers for their relationships with students.

- The curriculum for preservice teachers should include the study of legislation concerning ethical decision making and treatment. Furthermore this study should involve the historical context and the moral obligations of society that brought about the enactment.

- Teachers-in-training need to know that behaving in an ethical manner has positive societal value because a path of righteousness garners people's trust. Trust, a most basic human behavior, in turn is required for people to live together in an orderly and systematic manner.

- Knowing "What is the right thing to do in the education of deaf children?" is not a simple question. There are substantial differences of opinion based on experience and little conclusive research. Both realities complicate ethical decision making.

- Ethics education should be an integral part of all preservice programs for teachers of the deaf. Without being taught about ethics they may make teaching decisions that are ethically incorrect.
- Teachers trained in a program emphasizing signing regularly land jobs working in oral programs. Similarly, teachers accept positions in total communication programs even though they lack proficient signing skills. Obviously, even before direct instruction begins the ethical implication should be considered by those doing the hiring and those being offered the jobs.
- It is not uncommon for ethical decisions to involve a pitting of what is good for an individual versus what is good for a larger group.

Follow-up References or Suggestions

- An individual interested in becoming a teacher of the deaf should consider, among the other factors for choosing a program, the ethics education the various programs offer.

Ethical Questions for Consideration

- At present, training programs for teachers of the deaf are under pressure from both the "economic rationalization" experienced at colleges and universities, and the philosophical spin-offs from mainstreaming and integration. Is it possible that the topic of "ethics" is one aspect of the teacher-training curriculum that suffers most?
- Faculty intensive teacher training classes with low enrollments suffer most from financially pressured academic governors in one instance, whereas polar pro-integrationalists claim that regular teachers can do the job with proper support. Does this mean that ethics training must be concentrated in the basic teacher-training curriculum to ensure adequate attention and development?
- Observation of the education of deaf children frequently confirms that regular teacher training is inadequate when the complexities of language—both oral and visual—are concerned. Add to this the need for knowledge of specialized methods, curricula, and technology, and it is soon clear that regular teacher education is woefully inadequate for the education of many deaf children. Do you agree that a teacher of the deaf is always required for children with hearing losses?
- Is it true that we can only support specialized segregated educational settings if the cost-benefit studies show that this type of program is economical over some prescribed long-term period? What is the role of teacher-training programs in answering this question? Is it ethical to not participate in the quest?
- Putting aside the arguments of general education training versus specialized training in deafness—can the further refined specialization within deaf education be justified?

10

THOUGHTS AND PROJECTIONS

ROD G. BEATTIE

AUTHOR INTRODUCTION

I remain as I wrote in Chapter 1: Still honored to be a teacher and researcher with interests in deafness and education. Still interested in the preparation of those who want to work in this interesting world. Still keen to see the topic of ethics, deafness, and education explored.

A FEW QUOTES TO CONSIDER

Since the early days when I was collecting material on ethics, and then more recently as I worked with the contributing authors and their material, I have struggled with two somewhat polar thoughts. The first is that, "we are all going to hell in a hand-basket." The second reflected the wry title of an Erma Bombeck book, *The Grass Is Always Greener Over the Septic Tank.* The contents of one of my original ethics files with the title "Pithy Ethical Quotes" seemed to support these thoughts, and thus my slide into a psychological bipolar disorder seemed certain to have its genesis in my struggle with divergent ethical ideas.

My "hell in a hand-basket" thinking bubbled to the surface when I stumbled across this quote in Noble (1995)

> Science cannot stop while ethics catches up...
>
> Elvin Stackman; *Life,* January 9, 1950

I struggled with the Stackman's message. Must the ethics battle always be from the direction of mopping-up created dilemmas? Surely we can carry more hope than that.

Unfortunately, I found I was also pushed to the hellish side by this quote I found in Nix (1977, p. 317)

> I am in the right and you are in the wrong. When you are stronger, you ought to tolerate me. For it is your duty to tolerate truth. But when I am stronger, I shall persecute you, for it is my duty to persecute error.
>
> Lord Thomas B. Macaulay

Perhaps Lord Macaulay has a point, but "what's with the attitude" and those contrasted words: right—wrong; tolerate—persecute; truth—error? Harsh words nullifying gentler others. No, Lord Macaulay, your words do not help me feel hopeful either: They make my hellish hand-basket thoughts take devilish wings.

Thank heavens, however, for dialectual thinking—juxtaposed ideas. In my collection of pithy quotes—I also found those that showed that greener grass was possible. Cabot, well before Stackman, placed some hope in his quote I also found in Noble (1995, p. 92).

> Ethics and science need to shake hands.
>
> Richard Clarke Cabot, 1868–1939

But if my heart was to sing as I run barefoot through untended green grass, I could not have been happier with the seeds sowed by Spinrad and Spinrad (1979). They acknowledged that common wisdom is influenced by "recurrent tales of corruption in every aspect of modern life" and "that ethics are what each of us thinks should govern the other fellow" (p. 89). But they strongly asserted that

> [. . .] life today is infinitely more ethical in many respects than any previous age. We have simple created more and higher ethical standards than in the past. ... Indeed, there is room to believe that what seems to be a decline in ethics is actually a rise in acceptable standards. (p. 89)

INTRODUCTION

I started this book with many thoughts in my head. My motivation piqued because I knew I had many ethical concerns for deaf children, their families, and the educational experience they survived or endured. I had no pat answers, solutions, or suggestions. I hoped by exploring a host of topics with the help of knowledgeable people from different backgrounds and locations that I would gain a better grasp of the field and perhaps a better understanding of the questions that should be asked and answered.

Personally, I have learned a great deal from the exercise. Few things came quickly or easily. The hackneyed exercise expression of "no pain–no gain" fit. The opening chapter and even this one were a struggle, but I took heart that I heard parallel comments from many of the contributing authors. The short ethical quotes and dilemmas to consider—some used others abandoned—were perhaps the easiest tasks I set myself. I found I only needed to reflect on the material or people and places and the words spilled out. A bit of polish and there was another one. Other topics, however, were difficult. My good ideas and intentions, before too long, resembled the trail of Web pages I leave in my wake when I start an inadequately conceived Internet search. The words and sentences jerked along. I would have an idea, but that idea would stall as another popped into my head.

As the contributing authors returned their material to me I eagerly read it. I realized that the clichés of opening the exotic-sounding "Pandora's box" or the more mundane "can of worms" fit the experience. Did they give me answers, solutions, or suggestions? Yes a few, but in much greater abundance they gave me more questions, queries, and complications. This I suppose is okay. I know more than I knew before taking up the challenge of pulling this book together. If nothing else, others will have a basis to build something better. They can look at the cracks and faults. They can start with a better foundation. Build with better material. I look forward to reading their efforts.

Originally I thought I would be focusing most of this chapter on the summary of the work from the contributing authors. I came to believe that that was unnecessary. Rather, I would like to have the readers, thinkers, and writers focus some of their attention on a small collection of topics that seem to be still wanting. The material from the chapter authors convinced me that educators should embrace or re-embrace the idea of charters of rights and codes of ethics. Equally, I was convinced that we need to be very aware or reminded of two threats to the making of ethical decisions. Threats certainly painted here using a very wide brush—but threats nevertheless. First, the threat from media, and second, for want of a better description, the threat from tribal conflicts. The next point I wanted to raise in this chapter concerned the need for the discussion of ethics, deafness, and education to be extended to include the complete age range. Ethical issues also arise for school-age children and adolescents, young adults and their transition to postsecondary education or work, the middle-aged, the elderly. I have no doubt that their ethical dilemmas are just as serious as those described for younger children. Furthermore, these dilemmas may be rooted in earlier decisions taken during the age-span focused on in this book. The final thought I would like to introduce is the cost of "unethics."

ADDITIONAL THOUGHTS ON WHAT IS NEEDED

In the broader context of searching or striving for social justice, charters of rights and codes of ethics are common in developed countries and large organizations. Reference to these charters and codes is frequent in a variety of circumstances: professional duties, political activities, enacting legislation, applying legal rulings or sanctions. Sometimes the charters have extended names or titles that apply to whole nations or very large groups and concern citizenship, well-being, or civil rights. In contrast, there are also charters and bills that protect small groups.

In the first of the following sections I want to consider "charters" with reference to "smaller groups" or individuals. In the second, I would like to introduce ethical codes that protect those who are, or may not be in positions of power. I am interested in this area because I believe that others who are involved with the education of children with hearing impairments and their parents should be. Sadly, pertinent examples of charters, bills, and codes for these individuals (i.e., deaf or hard of hearing) are few or they have had limited circulation. (For general information on codes of ethics see the Web site of the Center for the Study of Ethics in the Professions at Illinois Institute of Technology. Available: http://csep.iit.edu/codes.)

Charters or Bills of Rights Concerning Speech/Language Impairments and Deafness

A simple search in the library and the Internet turned up one hit for a bill of rights for children with speech or language impairments, and a second focusing on deaf and hard of hearing children. Van Hattum (1985) outlined the five-point bill of rights for children with speech and language impairments. The points concerned the right to early screening and identification, in-depth evaluation, planned services, therapy provision, and prevention of complications. Rosen (1997) reported that a bill of rights for deaf and hard of hearing children has been increasingly proposed and enacted in separate states in the United States. The momentum for a bill of rights for the deaf arose from the Commission on Education of the Deaf (COED) report from 1988 that outlined the unsatisfactory status of deaf education and recommended specific changes. In 1992 a Deaf Child's Bill of Rights was presented for consideration of incorporation in the Education of the Deaf Act. Although the document was not incorporated in the Act at the time, it was later included, at least partially, in some states' legislation. In the Web page document, Rosen listed six states with enacted legislation and seven more with proposals for adoption.

Rosen (1997) highlighted the common provisions in all of these acts or bills, and also listed a collection of the unique provisions under the headings of "Communication," "Curriculum and Program Development," and "Services and Assistance by the Appropriate Educational Agency." Rosen stated the gist of the common provisions for deaf and hard of hearing children were:

- The children's ability to communicate is a priority.
- There must be qualified and certified personnel available who can communicate directly with the children.
- The children shall have an education with a sufficient number of same language mode peers who are of the same age and ability level.
- The children shall have opportunities to interact with deaf and hard of hearing adult role models.

- The children shall derive equal benefit from all services and programs at their schools.
- Assessment of children shall be appropriately administered.

Philosophically, few broad-minded people would quibble with these statements, but I suspect even the most optimistic would acknowledge that several would be impossible to achieve in most locations.

Alternative Charters or Bills of Rights

Unlike the charters or bills that carry the weight of law, some statements of rights are informal. Some time ago, while reading a student's logbook from their practice teaching experience, I found a photocopied page concerning rights of parents. I wondered where the student had found the sheet and I was sorry that my search for a reference was unsuccessful. The information, however, was interesting. On this page, the boxed title reminded us of the emphasis that our society places on rights, opportunities, and justice. The first two points concerned parents being given all the information about their child, and being able to make all the decisions for the child's future and placement. The last two points stated that the parents had the right to be involved in all discussions about their child, and that eventually the child, with maturity, has a right to participate in decisions that concern them.

This brief document went on to consider that parents' rights are also linked with supports. The first point stated that information not understood requires further explanation, and this legitimizes the parents asking questions. Second, unsatisfactory advice or service permits a parent to seek other advice elsewhere. And third, that parents have the right to seek out support and advocacy including that from other parents.

I was quite struck by this brief charter or bill of rights-like handout. In short order it had the potential to empower parents in a way that some extended discussions might not. Brief, yet useful. Powerful, but simple. I wondered why the author was not identified—my search continues.

In a somewhat similar format I found another charter or bill-like statement on a Web site designed by B. Penman that has subsequently disappeared or changed html address. In part, it reminded me of the recipes for a happy life or a good marriage that one finds in community cookbooks produced by service clubs. Pleasant enough, some food for thought—a degree of truth. I was moved again with the power of short documents. Essentially, the artistically arranged statements informed parents of their rights—the right to feel angry, to seek options, to set limits, to be enthusiastic. It also reminded parents, among other things, that they had a right to be annoyed, to have time off, and be treated with dignity (Penman, 1999, reprint from the FNDC Newsletter).

I mention these alternative charters and bills of rights mostly for consideration and discussion. Parents and teachers will find them or others just as I did. I recognize that some reflect enshrined legal points, but generally they remain at the commonsense level and are intended to be for moral support. Legal challenges abound for even the recognized bills of rights in different countries written by the "best" legal minds. And certainly, there is much that has not been scrutinized from a legal perspective in these alternative documents.

Codes of Ethics

I started my preliminary search for codes of ethics relating to exceptionalities from a personal point of reference: the *Code of Conduct for Research Involving Humans* prepared by the Tri-Council Working Group in 1996. Although this document concerned ethics for social-science researchers in Canada, it still highlighted many basic points relevant to education—and it was certainly useful in developing the Extended Glossary for this book. Branching out, I found a variety of codes for various professional groups: psychologists, speech-language pathologists and audiologists, auditory-verbal therapists, and teachers of exceptional children. Some of the codes, such as the Tri-Council document, are provided as a handout by the governmental research-funding body. Others appeared as appendixes in textbooks commonly used in university training courses. For example, Silverman's (1995) speech and language text reproduced the *Code of Ethics of the American Speech-Language-Hearing Association,* and Estabrooks's (1994) book included the *Professional Code of Ethics* developed by Auditory-Verbal International, Inc. for certified practitioners of auditory/verbal therapy. Still other codes were available on the Web sites of professional organizations. See for example, the *Council for Exceptional Children Code of Ethics and Standards of Practice (1997)* (CEC, 1999) or the *Canadian Code of Ethics for Psychologists (1991)* (CPA, 1999).

Codes for Professionals Who May Work with Children with Hearing Impairments

The Council for Exceptional Children's (CEC, 1999) *Code of Ethics and Standards of Practice (1997)* is an integrated document attempting to bridge or link the codes of ethics and the appropriate related standards of practice. The actual *Code of Ethics for Educators of Persons with Exceptionalities,* presented first is encapsulated in an opening declaration and eight principles. Although membership in the CEC by teachers and administrators is voluntary, the number of teachers of the deaf who hold membership is likely substantial, and may indeed be growing as smaller "independent" deafness-focused professional teaching organizations decline. For this reason alone it is worthwhile to include this general code of ethics for information purposes.

> We declare the following principles to be the Code of Ethics for educators of persons with exceptionalities. Members of the special education profession are responsible for upholding and advancing these principles. Members of The Council for Exceptional Children agree to judge and be judged by them in accordance with the spirit and provisions of this Code. (CEC, 1999)

After this opening statement eight points are listed. The first concerns a commitment to the highest quality education and development of quality-of-life potential.

The second addresses levels of competence and integrity in professional practice. The third focuses on engaging in professional activities that benefit individuals with exceptionalities, their families, other colleagues, students, and research subjects. The fourth and fifth points address objective professional judgment in professional practice and the advancement of professional knowledge and skills. Point six notes that professionals must work within the standards and policies of their profession, while the seventh notes the advocacy role for professionals to uphold and improve where necessary the laws, regulations, and policies governing the delivery of special education services. The eighth and last point concerns avoidance of unethical or illegal acts that violate adopted CEC professional standards (CEC, 1997).

The *Code of Ethics of the American Speech-Language-Hearing Association (1992),* although organized in a different fashion to that of the CEC, has a similar underlying purpose. That purpose is clearly stated in the preamble: "The preservation of the highest standard of integrity and ethical principles is vital to the successful discharge of the professional responsibilities of all speech-language pathologists and audiologists" (Silverman, 1995, p. 228).

In format "the fundamental rules of ethical conduct are described in three categories: Principles of Ethics, Ethical Proscriptions, Matters of Professional Propriety" (Silverman, 1995, p. 228). A total of "five Principles serve as a basis for the ethical evaluation of professional conduct and form the underlying moral basis for the Code of Ethics" (Silverman, p. 228). The Proscriptions are derived from the Principles of Ethics and are formal statements of prohibition. The "Matters of Professional Propriety represent guidelines of conduct designed to promote the public interest and thereby better inform the public and particularly the persons in need of speech language pathology and audiology services as to the availability and the rules regarding the delivery of those services" (Silverman, p. 228). In numerical sequence the ASHA Principles of Ethics for information sake are:

1. Individuals shall hold paramount the welfare of persons served professionally.
2. Individuals shall maintain high standards of professional competence.
3. Individuals' statements to persons served professionally and to the public shall provide accurate information about the nature and management of communicative disorders, and about the profession and services rendered by its practitioners.
4. Individuals shall honor their responsibilities to the public, their profession, and their relationships with colleagues and members of allied professions.
5. Individuals shall uphold the dignity of the profession and freely accept the profession's self-imposed standards. (Silverman, p. 228)

Features of Codes for Professionals Working with Children with Hearing Impairments

My basic search efforts turned up only one code of ethics for those who exclusively work with children with hearing impairments and their families. In this case, "those focusing on children with hearing impairments who have the potential to develop speech and language through the optimal use of amplified residual hearing" (Estabrooks, 1994, p. 295). Auditory-Verbal International Inc. (AVI) highlighted two features of the code in the preamble:

> This Professional Code of Ethics applies to those members who are responsible for the proper delivery of (re)habilitative services to such clients. The Professional Code of Ethics also seeks to protect persons served and to ensure the integrity of recognized auditory-verbal practices. (Estabrooks, p. 295)

AVI used a two-part structure for their professional code: Principles of Ethics and Rules of Ethics. From the preamble

> The Principles of Ethics, aspirational and inspirational in nature, form the underlying moral bases for the Professional Code of Ethics. Individuals shall observe these principles as affirmative obligations under all conditions of professional activity. Rules of Ethics are specific statements of minimally acceptable professional conduct or of prohibitions and are applicable to all individuals. (Estabrooks, p. 295)

The five Principles are then presented. The first, addressing agreement with the purpose, philosophy, and working principles of AVI and providing individuals with the practices that encourage habitual and maximal use of amplified residual hearing; second, honoring the paramount responsibility to the persons served professionally; third, honoring the "responsibility to achieve and maintain the highest level of professional competence" (Estabrooks, 1994, p. 295); fourth, honoring the "responsibilities to the public through providing information and education and the development of services for unmet needs" (Estabrooks, p. 295). And finally, honoring the

> [. . .] responsibilities to their own professionals, and maintain good relationships with, among others, AVI colleagues, members of allied professions, parents and students. Individuals shall uphold the dignity and autonomy of the professions, maintain harmonious interprofessional and intraprofessional relationships, and accept the professions' self-imposed standards. (Estabrooks, p. 295)

It is indeed unfortunate that more codes of ethics were not readily available so that the important points could be shared for the benefit of others. I will admit there are surely more codes available—unfortunately they have not been obvious or easy to find. I must applaud those profession organizations that have made theirs readily available.

SUPPORTS, THREATS, AND COMPLICATIONS

As the topics of ethics, childhood deafness, and education were brought together in the chapters of the contributing authors, other factors emerged—some stated directly in their text—others indirectly through our correspondence. The two factors I will feature here concern the effects of the media and influence of the tribal conflicts based in the history of deaf education. The impact from these factors, I believe, can range from highly positive to highly negative. My goal here is to present some thoughts and positions for consideration.

Media Support or Interference

The reporting of medical breakthroughs or advances has become a regular feature in the media. Coverage, in most instances, one would hope would have positive consequences. Regardless, the health reporter is now a specialty with almost every paper and television station. Their assignments are often reported in a formulaic fashion in regular time slots. Universities, medical research facilities, pharmaceutical companies, and the like are scoured for "newsworthy" items. In the visual-electronic media the talking-head shot of the health reporter opens the piece and continues to voice-over the segment. The video clip of an interviewed lab-coated doctor-figure is inserted first, followed by a cut-away to another lab-coated figure turning knobs on an impressive-looking instrument or using a scientific gewgaw (like the multi-ended pipette simultaneously depositing drops of colored liquid into rows of test tubes). To end the piece the reporter, staring directly into the camera, solemnly reports of untold numbers who could benefit and that clinical trials will start immediately although results and application are 5 to 10 years down the road.

On some unknown schedule each organ, disease, or affliction is given a turn by the reporters—ears being no different than eyes, lungs, or kidneys. A curmudgeon perhaps, but I believe the media have figured-out that articles and sound bites on ears and hearing are easily set up to help sell papers or increase ratings. Reporters and producers have realized there are divergent opinions or interests and a great deal of "emotional baggage" in the field of deafness. Claiming to know little, which may be true, the reporter's concept of delivering a balanced report is to juxtapose flaming remarks. Thus the balanced report consists of assembling the teams with opposing viewpoints. Yes, call me jaded if you will, but is this not a common approach for media pieces on deafness and language, educational methods, integration/mainstreaming, cochlear implants, and now hair-cell regeneration?

I have come to believe that this type of media coverage contributes little to the education and well-being of individuals with hearing impairments. I wonder if it actually educates the public or generates either interest or financial support for research. If there are positive outcomes from reporting emotional controversies, I would be willing to reevaluate my beliefs. In the meantime surely there are many other ways to positively portray individuals with hearing loss using different languages, diverse means of communication, and varied assistive-listening equipment. If, however, it is only the reporting of "failure" or "controversy" in deafness that brings attention or money, then I am truly saddened and ethically disappointed.

Tribal Conflicts

It is unfortunate that sarcastic names such as "Rabid Oralists, Sign Freaks, or Oral/Sign Nazis" are used to describe the very extreme positions of deaf education. The names exist because the groups exist. Are the names politically correct or socially acceptable? No! Are they widely known or used? Unfortunately yes. The extreme positions and the means by which they are expressed complicate the topic of deafness, ethics, and education. Often the innocent and naive are left more injured, confused, and ill informed than before they encountered the extremists. Ethically, morally, and emotionally this must be maltreatment.

The zealousness of hard-line fanatic in the field of deafness is remarkable. From observing and listening it seems they actually believe that they have "The Answer" to the problem of deafness. Their dialectic simplicity, things are black or things are white, is barely conceivable except at abstract or theoretical levels. If black, then do "x," if white, "y" is the solution. No gray, no complicating factors, no substantial differences, no doubt. One can only wish that deaf education was that simple!

It is interesting to ponder where the strength of these extreme convictions begins. Certainly as Moores (1996) intimates, research, what precious little there is of any quality in many areas, does not seem to form the basis of tribal positions and conflicts. In reality, it often appears that research, if used at all as a basis for a position, is that which was done by the holder of a position to support the position initially held. Similarly, any research that is counter the position held—if mentioned at all—is invariably discounted as inaccurate, unreliable, or biased. Hearing the honest answer to the simple question, "When was the last time you read a research paper supporting a position opposite your own?" could be quite revealing.

So returning to ponder the basis of extreme convictions, I am left to wonder how much we can ethically do to support parents and their children with hearing losses. Is our personal experience and convictions useful to the parents if we shared it with them? Perhaps! Or is the potential for bias too great? Possibly! Professionals cannot walk a mile in a parent's shoes. Parents, I am sure, do not want to walk a mile in ours. We cannot know others' experiences in all ways, and foreseeing the future is as much beyond us as claiming to have eliminated our personal biases. A right to influence the choices of others from claimed ethical and moral high ground is unfounded. Most, eventually, will surely call it meddling. Presenting available options, providing direction for additional information, providing moral support, and allowing decisions to be made without criticism or condemnation by those in the position to legally make the decisions is all that should be done.

PROJECTIONS FOR OLDER INDIVIDUALS WITH HEARING IMPAIRMENTS

As mentioned at the beginning of this chapter, I believe the discussion of ethics, deafness, and education should be extended: Not just the first 6 years, but also to school-age children, adolescents, young adults, and beyond. I am convinced that the people with hearing impairments in other age groups have both ongoing and unique educational needs with ethical overtones. I hope that the following brief discussion featuring several points will serve as a stimulus for others to take up the cause.

Some people may think that some of the issues that were discussed for children in the first 6 years are closed or "done-with" like bridges crossed and burned. This, however, seems unlikely from observation. Yes, the choice of first language may have been made when the child was an infant, but circumstances, attitudes, and choices change. Experience certainly exposes educators to parents and students who express doubt, concern, and even long-time resentment. As an individual with a hearing impairment ages, the first language choice made by the parents may be rejected by the deaf individual in favor of a later-acquired/desired language. Indeed, this choice may be made even though the person with the hearing loss is a very competent user of the first language chosen by the parents. This choice may be inspired by a host of reasons: friendship, perceived failure, comfort or ease, peer group pressure, marriage, educational choices, employment, and economic opportunities. Disregarding the individual rights perspective, I have heard people express disappointment or even condemnation over deaf individuals making this alternative language choice. Interestingly, the ethical question that might be posed is At what age does the deaf individual's choice supersede that of the parents—25, 21, 18, perhaps 12, or even 6? And following on this line of thinking then, At what age does a child's choice of education institution and method of instruction supersede that of the parents—12,16, 18, 21?

Another item for discussion that spans the educational experience of children with a hearing loss is the ethical appropriateness of integrated or mainstream placements. It is not difficult to understand the motivations behind this placement decision, including living with parents and family, exposure to the larger hearing society, and access to the same curriculum as hearing students, but what of the negatives or limitations? Finding the balancing point between the benefits of integration or mainstreaming and the real possibility of isolation and loneliness from a lack of teachers and peers as real communicative partners is a difficult task.

It is also during the later ages that a person with a hearing impairment must bear the ethical aspects of curriculum choices. The tolerable developmental delays in language and academic areas of young children may eventually force curriculum choices that have the effect of reducing the breadth or extent of the student's knowledge. What are the ethical implications of awarding a school-leaving certificate that may substantially misrepresent the knowledge and skills of the school-leaver relative to hearing peers? What are the ethical implications of this knowledge gap for students with hearing losses as they make the transition from school to work? How do we find the balance between the special admission requirements and affirmative action programs for spaces in training programs? What about the required funding of compensation programs for tertiary education facilities, training or apprenticeship programs, and ultimately employers?

COST OF UNETHICS

Unethics is a term I came across when Tim Banks used it in a 1999 article in *Management Today*. The adjective "unethical" was familiar—the novel "unethics" for me was new, but I did not need a definition. I recognized in an instant how it could apply to the topic of this book. In the same instance, however, I also saw how much more complex it was when we changed the perspective and context from that of management and organizations to that of well-being and quality of life for children with hearing losses. Certainly Banks reported that the "cost of unethical practices in Australian organizations are substantial and varied" (p. 19), but the illustrative examples highlighted moneys lost. Banks stated that the St. James Ethics Center, found "fraud cost the Australian economy in the region of $3.5 billion a year" and Morgan and Banks "found that 13% of the sick leave taken each year is not genuine, which costs employers about $2.5 billion" (p. 19).

Impressive as huge amounts of money may be in a discussion of "business" and unethics—I am left to ponder the question about the worth of individual humans. Odious as the thought may be of attaching a monitory value to an individual with a hearing loss for a life less lived because of unethical "educational" decisions—doesn't the struggle with this concept have value? We know unethical decisions for children with hearing impairments have consequences. The consequences include some that may be relatively easy to attach a monitory value to: the cost of "remedial" educational, chronic underemployment, even social assistance. However, how do we measure the worth of being unable to communicate with family or friends? What is the cost of not developing a child's cognitive skills to his or her potential? What value do we place on happiness and contentment missed? These, I believe need to be considered, but the quality-of-life research has miles to go in the area of unethics and the education of children with hearing losses.

CONSIDERING CLOSURE

Considering closure seems like the only reasonable thing for me to do with this book on ethics, deafness, and education. I believe declaring closure at this time is both inappropriate and impossible. I recognized that my purpose in this chapter was to widen the perspective of the book rather than attempt to condense and conclude both my own thinking and the work of the contributing authors. The authors surveyed, studied, sorted, and surely summarized their own work when they could. Continuing the alliteration, I am confident I could have added—"struggled." Of my own work, I know I have.

I am also well aware that much of this final chapter has no basis in research or scholarly review. This needs to be corrected. From experience, however, I had a strong suspicion that I would not have found the research I desired. I guess, in this last chapter I wanted not only to push myself but others as well. I wanted to show in the "what is needed" section that there are professions and organizations that have taken aspects of ethics seriously enough to produce bills of rights and codes of ethical conduct. Their efforts are valuable and should be seriously considered as models for drawing and sustaining the attention to this important topic. I believe, as I stated at the Chapter 1 that the topic of ethics in the field of deafness, hearing impairments, and deaf education has been overlooked or neglected. I hope others do follow-up research. I hope they extend, expand, challenge, and debate the material contained in these 10 chapters. Even more, I hope that topics and issues missed are taken up and not left to languish.

With open arms, and I hope with a similarly open mind, I welcome new thinking and contributions. Do not tarry. Bring it on. Test the waters as we have dared. I have no doubt that there are others, more ethics knowledgeable, ethics experienced, and ethics insightful than this person originally and proudly from Saskatchewan.

REFERENCES

American Speech-Language-Hearing Association. (1995). Code of Ethics of the American Speech-Language-Hearing Association (1992). In F. H. Silverman, *Speech, language, and hearing disorders* (pp. 228–238). Boston: Allyn Bacon.

Banks, T. (1999, June). A stitch in time: Organizations would do well to do good right now as ethics-to-go might give you heartburn. *Management Today,* 14–19.

Canadian Psychological Association. (1999). *Canadian Code of Ethics for Psychologists—Revised 1991* [On-line]. Available: http://www.cpa.ca:80/ethics.html.

Council for Exceptional Children (CEC). (1999). *CEC Code of Ethics and Standards of Practice (1997)* [On-line]. Available:http://www.cec.sped.org/ps/code.htm.

Estabrooks, W. (Ed.). (1994). *Auditory-verbal therapy for parents and professionals.* Washington, DC: Alexander Graham Bell Association for the Deaf.

FNDC Newsletter. (1999). Your rights as a parent. In B. Penman, *Children with a hearing loss: Parents rights* [On-line]. Found on: http://www.brandysign.com/rights.html.

Moores, D. F. (1996). *Educating the deaf: Psychology, principles, and practices* (4th ed.). Boston: Houghton Mifflin.

Nix, G. W. (Ed.). (1977). The rights of hearing-impaired children. *The Volta Review, 79*(5), 263–351.

Noble, K. A. (1995). *The international education quotations encyclopaedia.* Buckingham: Open University Press.

Rosen, S. (1997). *A synopsis of the Bill of Rights for Deaf and Hard of Hearing Children* [On-line]. Available: http://nad.policy.net/proactive/newsroom/release.vtml?id=17960.

Silverman, F. H. (1995). *Speech, language, and hearing disorders.* Boston: Allyn & Bacon.

Spinrad, L., & Spinrad, T. (1979). *Speaker's lifetime library.* Englewood Cliffs, NJ: Prentice-Hall.

Tri-Council Working Group. (1996). *Code of conduct for research involving humans.* Ottawa, ON: Minister of Supply and Services.

Van Hattum, R. J. (1985). *Organization of Speech-Language Services in the Schools: A manual.* Austin, TX: Pro-Ed.

APPENDIX

Important or Main Points

- Although a final chapter is often a summary and a chance to make recommendations, it can also be a "last chance" to touch on important topics that received less or little attention. This essentially was the nature of this final chapter.

- The topic of charters of rights and codes of ethics has received attention in a number of areas relating to deafness or hearing impairments. The degree of formality of the charters or codes varies. The familiarity of professionals to charters and codes will likely be highly variable.
- The role that the media can play was discussed—in particular how the "balanced-report" of some topics may simply be a means for attracting an audience or increasing ratings.
- The age-old methods debates have not abated in many instances. These often emotionally based debates can fuel ongoing ethical dilemmas.
- There should be a discussion of ethics and education of individuals with hearing losses that considers the life span.
- There is a "cost" for unethical behavior. It may be possible to attach a monetary value in some instances, but many of the human dimensions defy simple "dollar" assignments.

Follow-up References or Suggestions

- Children's Defense Fund. (1992). *The state of America's children 1992.* Washington, DC: Author.

    Although not focused on deafness and ethics, the general material in this report is interesting reading in its discussion of comparisons of cost of prevention to costs of supports.

- Cheng, A. K. et al. (2000). Cost-utility analysis of the cochlear implant in children. *Journal of the American Medical Association, 284*(7) [On-line]. Available: http://jama.ama-assn.org/issues/v284n7/rfull/joc00352.html. This paper is an interesting deafness-related example where the objective of the authors was "to determine the quality of life and cost consequences for deaf children who receive a cochlear implant."

Ethical Questions for Consideration

- Effective means for educating professionals about codes of ethics is important. Where and when should this occur?
- Should national organizations of the deaf consider establishing media guidelines for ethical reporting of stories?
- What is the time or age when a deaf individual is partially or wholly responsible for making a contribution or contributing to the decision making relative to the content and means of their own education, work training, employment, and living arrangements?
- Is it possible to put a priority on a collection of educational ethical issues with consideration to such things as age of deaf individual or the language of

the family? Or is the nature of ethics, deafness, and education so varied that global priorities are impossible?

- What is the role for educators in the discussion of ethical issues concerning quality of life and cost consequences?
- Is it possible to prioritize future research topics in the ethics area?

EXTENDED GLOSSARY

Advocacy   Reynolds and Fletcher-Janzen (1990) believe that the term advocacy "has a variety of meanings, depending on who is providing the advocacy. In its essence, advocacy refers to attempts by an individual handicapped person, by another person, or by a group to guarantee that all rights due a handicapped person are realized" (p. 42). Later, citing Bateman (1982) Reynolds and Fletcher-Janzen caution that "individual special educators acting alone or through professional organizations, may also view themselves as advocates for the handicapped children they serve, [but] there may be inherent conflicts in attempting to play the two roles simultaneously" (p. 42). Williams (1991) also clarifies the term advocacy by noting that the role "is distinguished from that of the expert witness, who gives a professional judgement and from that of the named person, who is essentially a counsellor and adviser" (p. 11).

Advocate   Two similar definitions are given in Merriam-Webster's *New Collegiate Dictionary* for "advocate" 1: one that pleads the cause of another: one that pleads the cause of another before a tribunal or judicial court, 2: one that defends or maintains a cause or proposal. Thus, a parent can and usually is an advocate for his or her child's best interests. It is also possible that in some instances a non-related adult becomes an advocate for another adult because of problems communicating in a second language.

Autonomy of Persons and Informed Decision Making (Principle of)   A dictionary definition of autonomy would concern an individual being self-governing. Thus follows the extended discussion from the Roeher Institute in cooperation with Inclusion International (1999)…

> Every person has the right to be independent and to make their own decisions. This includes the right, based on free and informed decisions, to receive or refuse medical treatment, health-care measures, research interventions, or knowledge of one's genetic characteristics. It also includes the right to have full information about the risks and benefits of

---

choices, to be told what alternatives and options are available, and to be supported in one's decisions. (WFD News, May 2000, p. 6)

Bias (Measurement/Test)   Tittle (1997) in simple language, states that: "To say a test is biased is to charge that it is prejudiced or unfair to groups or individuals characterized as different from the majority of test takers" (Keeves, 1997, p. 813). Earlier, Hardman, Drew, Egan, and Wolf (1993) used a longer definition describing test bias as the "error introduced during testing when a procedure or test instrument gives one group a particular advantage or disadvantage" and "usually involves factors unrelated to ability, such as culture, gender, and race" (p. 491).

Beneficence   In simple terms beneficence involves doing or producing good to or for others. The Merriam-Webster's dictionary expands this basic definition by adding, "performing acts of kindness or charity." The Tri-Council (1996) uses research as an example for describing beneficence and the potential good research produces. First, there is good for society as a whole, including the general production of knowledge. Second, there is good for the research subjects; and third, there is good for the researchers, their sponsors, and institutions. The Tri-Council, however, counsels that the presence of helping professionals in research projects may be problematic because they may carry with them "the explicit or implicit promise of benefit to the research subject" (p. 2–3).

Casuistry/Case-Based Reasoning   Kuczewski (2000) states that the "casuists are similar to the principlists in holding that medical ethics involves applying role-specific morality to the circumstances of particular cases. However, the casuists emphasize even more strongly how important the particular circumstances are for the proper resolution of problematic cases" [On-line]. To solve a complex ethical problem the casuist will look for similar but clearer cases with different solutions. These simpler cases, then, by analogy, should point-out the "better" solution depending on which of the alternatives the complex case most resembles. (Kuczewski suggests Albert R. Jonsen, 1991, or Carson Strong, 1988, as sources for additional information.)

Categorical/Noncategorical System/Approach   In special education, a categorical system or approach is a classification system that uses specific categories such as learning disabilities or mental retardation to identify groups of people. The noncategorical system or approach involves "not classifying or differentiating among disabilities in providing services" (Smith, Luckasson, & Crealock, 1995, p. 9). (For a discussion of positive and negative attributes for both systems, see Smith et al., 1995.)

Clinical Trial(s)   Merriam-Webster's dictionary defines clinical trial as a tryout or experiment to test quality, value, or usefulness of something like a drug or procedure. The second part of the definition states that the trial is generally one of a number of repetitions of an experiment to ensure that the same or similar result is found each time. Pocock (1983) as cited by the Tri-Council (1996) reports that,

> [. . .] there is an ever-increasing number of treatment innovations which require proper investigation to see if they are of genuine benefit to patients. The randomized controlled clinical trial has become widely regarded as the principal method for obtaining a reliable evaluation of treatment effects on patients. (Section 18)

Code of Ethics   Reynolds and Fletcher-Janzen (1990) cite Fisher (1978) who defined a code of ethics as "the formal, well established standards that a profession follows in order to protect and promote the welfare of its clients and society" (p. 116). Similarly, they cite Paul (1981) who says the "prime responsibility of special educators lies in ensuring that the individuals they serve receive the services they need and are granted their educational rights" (p. 413). Keith-Spiegel and Koocher (1985) do add a note of caution however, because a genuine commitment to protecting the interest of persons served is only one reason for developing a code of ethics. The second reason concerns the self-interests of the profession or its members to protect themselves in possible situations of malpractice or incompetence by a fellow member.

Communitarian Bioethics Kuczewski (2000) reports that communitarian bioethics "is an offshoot of a larger political and social movement pioneered by philosophers such as Alasdair MacIntyre, Michael Sandel, and Charles Taylor" [On-line]. These philosophers and others "believe that the problem in ethics and politics is that the U.S. is a pluralistic society in which few values are shared. This lack of shared values leaves us with sparse conceptual resources with which to discuss ethical problems." To correct the situation, the thinkers believe it necessary to restore "some shared hierarchy of goods or common values" through genuine dialogue in smaller community-based units. (Kuczewski suggests Ezekiel J. Emanuel, 1992, as a source for additional information.)

Confidentiality In simple terms confidentiality is about keeping sensitive information private or secret. In education, Hallahan and Kauffman, (1991) state that "the results of evaluations and placement must be kept confidential, though the child's parents or guardians may have access to the records" (p. 25). Williams (1991) adds that confidentiality is:

> [. . .] an ethical principle that has caused considerable concern. Some sensitive information about a child's background and development may be essential for a thorough understanding of his or her needs, yet a parent may volunteer the information without wishing it to be passed on. In this situation, if persuasion is unsuccessful, confidences must be respected. (p. 91)

(For an extended discussion on this topic with research studies see the Tri-Council, 1996.)

Conflict of Interest Merriam-Webster's definition of a conflict of interest focuses on the conflict between the private interests and the official responsibilities of a person in a position of trust. The dictionary suggests, as an example, a government official, who may be may be responsible for policy development and those policies will be personally beneficial in a financial sense. In the area of deafness, conflicts of interest could arise in many areas. A simple example could be a private audiologist recommending a hearing aid—not because it is the best instrument for the client, but rather it represents one that the clinician receives the highest sales commission from the manufacturer.

Consequentialism Consequentialism is a traditional ethical theory that argues that actions are good or bad based depending upon their consequences. Kuczewski (2000) states that "the best-known form of consequentialism is called utilitarianism, a position that claims we need to take the actions that generally lead to happiness or pleasure" [On-line]. Kuczewski reports that consequentialists try to form basic rules to guide their action. As an example, Kuczewski cites the general rule of "Choose the action that is likely to produce the greatest good for the greatest number." (See Kuczewski's follow-up recommendation of Kagan (1989) who reports on the works of John Stuart Mill and Jeremy Bentham.)

Consent/Informed Consent Singh and Powers (1993) in describing helping relationships, wrote that: "Informed consent is much more than a simple legal procedure. It represents a general principle for working with families" (p. 21). Listed obligations for consent include (a) safeguarding the privacy and autonomy, (b) ensuring that family members are willing participants, and (c) that purpose and goals are clearly stated, understood, and found satisfactory. For research, the Tri-Council (1996) featured other important comments about informed consent. For example: "Free consent is uncoerced consent," and "It is also important that, whenever possible, potential research subjects be given adequate time and privacy to reflect on their participation in the research protocol" (p. 2–9). (See the Tri-Council 1996 document for additional information on subject-centered perspective and consent.)

Continuing Ethical Review   An ongoing or continuing ethical review has its basis in research. The Tri-Council (1996) identifies both the purpose and important issues:

> The first term of reference for REBs [Research Ethics Boards] is the protection of research subjects from research harms. Having said this, it is important to appreciate why the continuing ethical review process is essential. Three issues are of particular importance to REBs: Drifting from a given protocol with maleficent intent; failure to comply with the intent of the initial protocol; and evaluation of possible changes in the probability and magnitude of harms that subjects may actually suffer. (Section 8)

Deinstitutionalization   Deinstitutionalization, originally the moving of individuals with mental retardation out of residential institutions to community living arrangements, was an outcome of the "normalization" philosophy that originated in Scandinavia in the 1950s and 1960s. Hallahan and Kauffman (1991) added that: "Deinstitutionalization requires not only moving people out of institutions but also having specific plans to integrate them into more normal community residences" (p. 64). Unfortunately, the lack of specific plans is often what appears lacking.

Deontology   A traditional ethical theory that is duty-based. Kuczewski (2000) states that: "The goal of [deontological] ethics is thought to be the fulfillment of one's duties or the carrying out of obligations without regard to one's desires" [On-line]. As Kuczewski continues, "because this school is suspicious of desire or happiness as a guide to moral action, deontologists usually seek a general basis for the duties such as an a priori principle (a principle which need not appeal to one's experience)" [On-line]. (See Kuczewski's recommendations of Kant (1996) and Rawls (1971) for the most commonly-cited formulations of the deontological approach.)

Dignity of Persons—Dehumanization   Although focused on research the 1996 Tri-Council ethics document defines dignity of person—dehumanization through examples. The description states that dehumanization occurs when,

> [. . .] one is afraid of physical and moral pain. One is afraid of losing one's freedom; of losing self-control; of being obliged to act against one's values; of having one's body degraded; or of being humiliated for one's personal history; or of having one's cultural or group identity mocked. (p. 1–5)

Dehumanization also occurs when,

> [. . .] one is afraid of others' prejudices; of seeing oneself or one's group reflected back in a negative light. One is afraid of acts or processes which might destabilize or disrupt one's inner equilibrium. One is afraid of being manipulated (physically or psychologically), of being transformed profoundly or irrevocably. (p. 1–5)

(See Tri-Council, 1996, for information relative to research and dehumanization.)

Dignity of Risk   Smith et al. (1995) report that dignity of risk refers to the situation where "students with disabilities are overprotected, deprived of the ordinary risks and challenges necessary for human development and essential to growing up. Students with disabilities should be allowed the dignity of risk to succeed or fail like others" (p. 21). "The principle of normalization as well as the principle of dignity of risk (Perske, 1972, in Wolfensberger, 1972) helped provide a foundation for the civil rights cases tried in the courts" (Smith et al., 1995, p. 129).

Diversity (Principle of)   The Roeher Institute in cooperation with Inclusion International (1999) as reprinted in the WFD News (2000, May) state

> The principle of diversity considers the population in terms of gender, race, religion, functional capacity, sexual orientation, and so on. Diversity implies not a goal of creating better people, but one of making a better world for all of us to live in. Thus diversity rejects technology such as prenatal diagnosis, gene probes, and gene therapy as a means of ridding the world of those who do not meet society's notions of "normality" or "perfection." (p. 6)

Due Process/Due Process Hearing   It is common that legislation for the provision of special education includes the right to due process through a due process hearing. Hallahan and Kauffman (1991) state that the "child's and parents' rights to information and informed consent must be assured before the child is evaluated, labeled, or placed, and they have a right to an impartial due process hearing if they disagree with the school's decisions" (p. 25). In the due process hearing the complainant's "rights include the right to legal counsel and other rights concerning witnesses, written evidence, verbatim documentation of the hearing, and an appeal" (Smith et al., 1995, p. 20).

Ethic(s)   Jacob-Timm and Hartshorne (1994) record that:

> The term *ethics* generally refers to a system of principles of conduct that guide the behavior of an individual. *Ethics* comes from the Greek *ethos,* meaning "character" or "custom," and the phrase *ta ethika,* which Plato and Aristotle used to describe their studies of Greek values and ideals. ... The terms *ethics* and *morality* are often used interchangeably. However, according to philosophers, the term *morality* refers to a subset of ethical rules of special importance. (p. 2)

> (See Solomon (1984) in Jacob-Timm & Hartshorne, 1994, for a development and clarification of the terms morality and ethics.)

Ethics and Special Education   Reynolds and Fletcher-Janzen (1990) outline a key list of ethical issues important for special educators.

> Special education professionals are responsible for knowing the ethical standards of the profession and must be knowledgeable about the rights of exceptional children and their parents. Parents of special education children need to be informed of these rights, including the granting of consent for evaluation, diagnosis, and education. The right to privacy of the individual youngster and the family must be protected and all records and pertinent information kept confidential. When delivering an intervention, special education professionals are mainly responsible for choosing an educational alternative that would not be harmful, physically or mentally, to the handicapped youngster. (p. 413–414)

Eugenics (Concerns)   The original popular movement of the late nineteenth and early twentieth centuries "concerned improving the genetic characteristics of a species, originally through selective breeding" (Williams, 1991, p. 159). Reynolds and Fletcher-Janzen (1990) discussed the link between breeding success with plants and animals and humans: "The idea of improving the human stock arose from the observation of the great diversity of human characteristics and abilities and the tendency for characteristics to run in families" (p. 418). Ultimately this movement led, in some places, to laws restricting marriage, institutional confinement, and sterilization. (See Tri-Council, 1996, for information clarifying the aim of contemporary genetic research versus the historical goals of eugenics.)

Exclusion and/or Exploitation (in Research)   Those with disabilities, along with minors, women, subordinate groups, prisoners, and others, are at special risk for being excluded and/or exploited in research endeavors. Concerning exploitation, the Tri-Council (1996) states: "While it would be paternalistic to conclude that no members of such groups can consent to participation, it is clear that there may be a need for special measures to ensure that consent is genuinely uncoerced" (p. 2–8). Alternatively, exclusion from participation in research may deny the individuals or groups from the benefits of research advances. (See Tri-Council, 1996, for additional information.)

Fairness   There is direct connection between fairness and ethics. Indeed, fairness will be a critical factor for every ethical decision. As Parashar (1977) wrote for the topic of assessment—fairness is:

> One of the essential qualities of an examiner, test material, and other variables which permits equal treatment to all the subjects involved. This quality reflects impartiality, absence of favors or prejudices, and freedom from the influence of strong feelings and personal bias. (p. 43)

Four Principles Approach/Principlism   Kuczewski (2000) describes this approach as a one "method" for operationalizing, in particular cases, the general nature of the theories of deontology, consequentialism, and virtue ethics. To do so, medical ethicists work with the mid-level vocabulary principles of respect for patient autonomy, beneficence, non-maleficence, and justice. Kuczewski states:

> Advocates of the four principles approach claim that doing medical ethics is a matter of balancing the four principles of autonomy, beneficence, non-maleficence, and justice in each case. Each of these four duties is always in effect but clinical ethical dilemmas can pit one of these duties against another. For example a case in which an acutely ill patient with a treatable condition wishes to refuse treatment and be allowed to die brings a conflict between respect for the patient's autonomy and the physician's duty of care for the patient's well-being (beneficence) [On-line]. (See Beauchamp & Childress, 1994, for additional information.)

Gene Therapy   A simple dictionary definition of gene therapy is: "the insertion of normal or genetically altered genes into cells usually to replace defective genes especially in the treatment of genetic disorders" (see Merriam-Webster's). Wolff-Heller, Alberto, Forney, and Schwartzman (1996) expanded the definition of gene therapy by adding, "the aim of gene therapy may include correcting certain cells to function normally by replacing the affected gene by its healthy counterpart or adding the healthy counterpart to the affected gene" (p. 293).

Genetic(s)   It is possible to combine the definitions of genetics by Reynolds and Fletcher-Janzen (1990) and Williams (1991) to provide one simple definition: Genetics is the science or study of the transmission of hereditary characteristics; this also includes the study of the variation of inherited characteristics. Williams makes two points concerning genetics and special education. First, "some of the conditions of which special education is required are carried by a single faulty gene ... whereas others are polygenic, caused by the interaction of several genes," and second, although genetics may not have "direct implications for educational procedures, its application will result in limiting the number of children born with special needs" (p. 181–182).

Genetic Counseling   Genetic counseling is primarily a specialized family planning activity, concerned with investigating the presence or possibility of a wide variety of traits or abnormalities, by a trained geneticist. To establish presence or possibility of a genetic trait, the geneticist will collect an extensive family history, conduct physical examinations, and/or employ a variety of laboratory tests—cytogenetic or biochemical analyses of cells, amniotic fluid, blood, etc. The conclusions from these studies then guide the counselor to inform the individuals. (See Northern & Downs, 1984, or Reynolds & Fletcher-Janzen, 1990 for additional information.)

Genetic Engineering   Mosby's dictionary of medical, nursing, and allied health terms described genetic engineering as the,

> [. . .] process of producing recombinant DNA so that the genotype and phenotype of organisms can be altered and controlled. Emzymes are used to break the DNA molecule into fragments so that genes from another organism can be inserted and the nucleotides rearranged in any desired sequence. (p. 514)

Although application in humans is still quite limited, eliminating malformations or possibly controlling genetic disorders is anticipated in the future.

Genome/Human Genome (Project)   A genome refers to one "haploid" set of chromosomes with the genes they contain. Broadly, genome means all the genetic material of an organism, whereas haploid refers to having the gametic number of chromosomes (i.e., number of chromosomes in the spermatozoon or ovum) or half the number characteristic of somatic cells. The human genome project is the multinational effort to develop/record the complete sequence of genes of one set of human chromosomes.

Genotype/Phenotype   A simple dictionary definition of genotype is "all or part of the genetic constitution of an individual or group"; in contrast, the definition of phenotype is "the visible properties of an organism that are produced by the interaction of the genotype and the environment" (Merriam-Webster's). Parashar (1977) extended the genotype description to include the "genetic constitution of an individual or combinations of inherited traits, conditions, characteristics, and dispositions. The overall effect of one's characteristics descended from ancestors irrespective of environmental influences" (p. 46).

Handicappism   Reynolds and Fletcher-Janzen, (1990) report that

> Handicapism is a term created by Bilken and Bogdan (1976) to identify both an evolving social movement and a set of behaviors toward those with disabilities. It has been defined by its authors as "a theory and set of practices that promote unequal and unjust treatment of people because of apparent or assumed physical or mental disability" (p. 9). ... Like racism and sexism, handicapism is evident in the language often used to describe disabled individuals. Such language tends to be discriminatory and serves to devalue the capabilities of the person (Heward & Orlansky, 1984; Mullins, 1979). (p. 494)

Human Genetic Research   The branch of biology dealing with the study of the phenomena of heredity and the laws governing it in humans. The Tri-Council (1996) uses the following phrasing: "Human genetic research involves the study of genetic factors (and the interaction of such factors with the environment) responsible for human traits, both normal and abnormal" (p. 15-1). (See Wolff Heller, Alberto, Forney, & Schwartzman, 1996, p. 390 for additional information on genetics and people with disabilities.)

Incentives for Participation   To have ethical research the Tri-Council (1996) noted that "the altruism that ideally underlies the enterprise of research is negated when the participation of a research subject is induced primarily by the promise of reward (in money or in kind, such as in free medical care)" (p. 10-2). While much educational research does not "offer" incentives for participation, there may be facets where there is application. For example, there may be the possibility of attending/enrolling in a particular educational program and thereby receiving specialized treatment or services.

Inclusion/Full Inclusion   Smith et al. (1995) define inclusion as the "practice of assuring that all students with disabilities participate with other students in all aspects of school" (p. 23 and 526). As a further development of the inclusion concept some proponents will use the term "full inclusions" and by this they support the "interpretation that states that the least restrictive environment for all children with disabilities is in the regular education classroom" (Smith et al., p. 82). In this definition extra emphasis is placed on the word "all."

Individualized (Educational/Family Service) Plans   An Individualized Plan, in one of several possible forms, is a "requirement that guarantees a specifically tailored program to meet the individualized needs of each student with disabilities" (Smith et al., 1995, p. 20). The educational plan or "IEP must include a statement of present educational performance, instructional goals, educational services to be provided, and criteria and procedures for determining that the instructional objectives are being met" (Hallahan & Kauffman, 1991, p. 481). An IFSP is the plan "to ensure that services for infants and toddlers under age 3 are provided in the context of the family" (Hallahan & Kauffman, p. 481). (See Hallahan & Kauffman, 1991, or Smith et al., 1995 for additional information.)

Integration   Hallahan and Kauffman (1991) provide a rather long but plain-English definition of integration:

> Integration is the normalization of where and with whom people with disabilities live, work, go to school, and play. Like other aspects of normalization, integration as a broadly supported social issue began in the 1960s. Integration involves the movement of people with disabilities from institutions to community living, from special schools to regular public schools, and from special classes to regular classes. (p. 53)

Restating this, Hallahan and Kaufman say, "integration means people with disabilities living, working, playing, and going to school with nondisabled people" (p. 64).

Justice/Justice (Principle of)

> The principle of justice upholds the rights and equality of individuals and groups. It affirms fairness and equality in the allocation of resources: all people have the right to develop their potential and to be provided with what is needed to achieve individual and social well-being. It rejects economic efficiency and cost effectiveness as ethical principles, and beneficence and best interest as the sole basis of government obligation. (Roeher Institute, 1999 cited in WFD News, 2000, p. 6)

The Tri-Council (1996) adds,

Justice is the ethical principle the law aims to serve. Conduct is not necessarily ethical because it is legal. Similarly, conduct that can be justified ethically is not necessarily legal, such as research beneficial for children in general that would expose individual child subjects to risk. (p. 2-3)

Justinian Code   Turkington and Sussman (1992) indicate that "all of Roman law as codified, including the legal rights of deaf citizens (which were basically nonexistent)" during the reign of Justinian I from A.D. 527–565 (p. 110). This very early document reflected aspects of the ethical treatment of those with hearing impairments. It indicated that "deaf Romans could not marry, and legal guardians were appointed to handle their affairs," but the code was more lenient for those with acquired deafness (p. 110). Indeed, if they could write they could handle their own affairs.

Labeling   In special education, labeling consists of assigning of a name or category to an individual, usually or often reflective of a physical or mental disability or behavioral characteristic. Hearing or vision impaired, mentally retarded, or behaviorally disordered are labels used to categorize people. Labels may be formally or informally given. Psychologists may formally impose a label of "learning disabled" after a battery of intellectual and educational assessments. Children in the playground may informally give the label of "dummy" to another child who struggles with academic material. Formal labels have the benefit of providing a common language to describe a disability and in some cases delivering financial support. Unfortunately, the same label may be harmful because it potentially degrades, discriminates, or excludes the individual. (See Reynolds & Fletcher-Janzen, 1990, for additional information.)

Least Restrictive Environment   Williams (1991) notes that least restrictive environment is a "phrase used in the USA to give effect to the principle that children with special needs should be educated in surroundings as normal as possible" (p. 245). Williams suggests that least restrictive environment is used in place mainstreaming because it "provides more flexibility, and allows a number of possibilities to be examined by the team of professionals and parents involved in deciding placement" (p. 245). Smith et al. (1995) suggest this flexibility allows for the philosophical position like that articulated in the Special Education Report (1992) "that residential schools for the deaf may be the least restrictive environment for many deaf children" (p. 456). (Also see Smith et al., 1995, for additional information.)

Legislation   Legislation concerns bills that become laws when passed by federal, provincial, state, or territorial government. Legislation in many areas may have an impact on ethical matters concerning individuals with disabilities. Some of the most likely legislation to raise ethical questions includes the areas of education, health, social services, employment, and immigration.

Litigation   Litigation involves a lawsuit or legal proceeding. The results of litigation may have an impact on many ethical matters. Like legislation, litigation may have a focus or a connection to the provision of education, health, social services, employment, and immigration services. The lawsuit may have at its basis a desire for compensation for correction of opportunities lost, services owed by not received, financial loss, or compensation for emotional and physical distress.

Mainstreaming   Hallahan and Kauffman (1991) simply define mainstreaming as "the integration of students with disabilities into general education classes" (p. 64). Turkington and Sussman (1992) have refined this definition for students with hearing losses suggesting mainstreaming is the "process in which a student with hearing problems attends some—or all—classes in a regular school for hearing students" (p. 110). Williams (1991) comments that mainstreaming "is the application of the principle of normalization to the educational system" (p. 254).

Morals   Merriam-Webster's *New Collegiate Dictionary* provides multiple definitions to the word moral or morals: "(1a) of or relating to principles of right and wrong in behavior; (1b) expressing or teaching a conception of right behavior; (1c) conforming to a standard of right behavior; (1d) sanctioned by or operative on one's conscience or ethical judgment; (1e) capable of right and wrong action." The follow-on definitions include: "(2) probably though not proved; (3) of, relating to, or acting on the mind, character, or will." Relative to discussion of ethics in this book the first five variations are most apt.

Named Person   Williams (1991) indicated that a named person was a "role proposed in the Warnock Report for an individual who could serve as a guide to parents of children with special educational needs" (p. 280). Williams reported that the named person would be a link between the family and professionals. Other activities may include accompanying parents to interviews, and making follow-up visits to ensure that procedures were understood. The named person may also suggest what help or advice the parents would find useful and then direct them to it if necessary.

Narrative Bioethics   Following his brief synopsis of theories and methods in bioethics, Kuczewski (2000) concluded that, "much of the work in bioethics depends upon constructing the case or issue such that its salient features come to the fore. ... As a result, some argue that behind each bioethics method is a kind of narrative activity" [On-line]. Kuczewski suggests that these narratives in bioethics are a promising avenue of inquiry and may remain so for some time. (See Kuczewski, 2000, [On-line] for additional information.)

Noncategorical Approach   In reference to special education a noncategorical approach means *not* grouping or classifying individuals on the basis of type of disability or the specialized services that may be provided. Parashar (1977) states that "a *Non-Categorical Approach* concentrates on the problem—learning, behavior or both—instead of labels of the child. In this approach the labels are discarded, and the diagnosis starts with identifying the problems" (p. 18). In contrast, the *Categorization Approach* places children or adults in classes or groups with labels like mentally retarded, emotionally disturbed, or learning disabled. Usually the label and grouping stems from the main exceptionality and relates to the individual's care, therapy, remediation, or education. (See Smith et al., 1995 for additional information.)

Nondiscrimination (Principle of)   From the Roeher Institute in cooperation with Inclusion International (1999): "The principle of non-discrimination is founded on the belief that everybody has the right to life, to medical treatment, and to acceptance without discrimination based on the existence or expectation of mental or physical disability, or any other characteristic" (Snoddon, 2000, p. 6). (See the Roeher Institute, 1999 for additional information.)

Nondiscriminatory Evaluation/Testing.   Relative to proper ethical behavior in the evaluation or testing of an individual with a disability, the examiners must adhere to nondiscriminatory criteria. First, to be nondiscriminatory, the individual's language, cultural characteristics, or handicaps should not bias the results. Second, any evaluation or testing for placement or planning must be made by a multidisciplinary team that does not rely on a single evaluation instrument or procedure. And finally, the assessment must be comprehensive—considering all areas that may be affected by the individual's disability. (See Hallahan & Kauffman, 1991, or Smith et al., 1995 for additional information.)

Nonmaleficence   Not harming others (Tri-Council, 1996, p. 1-1). Further, nonmaleficience or the principle of nonmalificence, "is interpreted in light of the principle of autonomy and in terms of the harm/benefit ratio. … Not harming can be extended in some circumstances to an obligation to prevent and even remove harm caused by others" (p. 2-2). For many people, nonmaleficence has a prohibitory moral flavor. This prohibition includes refraining from actions that harm, injure, or otherwise violate the basic rights of individuals. (Consult the documentation of an appropriate ethics research committee for further information.)

Normalization   Hallahan and Kauffman (1991) outlined the origin, dissemination, and description of normalization in one sentence: "First espoused in Scandinavia and later popularized in the United States by Wolfensberger (1972), [normalization] is the philosophical belief that every person with a disability should have an education and living environment as close to normal as possible" (p. 40). Williams (1991) added a useful expansion, stating that normalization espouses "the belief that persons with handicaps should enjoy the same privileges, rights and opportunities as persons without handicaps" (p. 289). (See Hallahan & Kauffman, 1991, for additional information.)

Privacy   In a discussion of ethics privacy is usually concerned with a variation of the dictionary definition of "freedom from unauthorized intrusion." As examples in general ethics, the right to privacy includes having personal information given for an assessment or evaluation kept confidential. It also means that the results of an assessment are treated with the same degree of confidentiality. There are many other references to the provision of privacy when individuals are concerned.

Provision of Service (Array/Continuum/Cascade)   An "array of service" refers to "a constellation of services, personnel, and educational placements … the system must respond to the needs of these students rather than force them into a rigid system." A "continuum of service" is "a graduated range of educational services; one level of service leads directly to the next one." The "cascade of services" is "a linear and sequential model used to describe educational environments from the most of the least restrictive" (Smith et al., 1995, p. 71). The link with ethics, then, is decision making and provision of the best educational placement for a child.

Rationality   Merriam-Webster's *New Collegiate Dictionary's* first three definitions for "rationality" were: (1) the quality of state of being rational, (2) the quality or state of being agreeable to reason, and (3) a rational opinion, belief, or practice. For ethical decision making the distinction between making a good or bad decision may hinge on whether it was made by a rational or irrational person or a rational process of thinking.

Respect for Persons   In research, this phrase concerns treating individuals with dignity and respect. Most research ethics review committees highlight two fundamental aspects of respect for persons.

> Respect for autonomy, which requires that those who are capable of deliberation about their personal choices should be treated with respect to their capacity for self-determination; and ... Protection of persons with impaired or diminished autonomy, which requires that those who are dependent or vulnerable be afforded security against abuse. (Tri-Council, 1996, p. 2-2. Also see this document for additional information.)

Responsibility for Adverse Outcomes   In research there is a collective and ethical responsibility on the part of the sponsor, the institution, the research ethics board, and the researcher to ensure that provisions are in place to meet legal liabilities for injuries or losses suffered by research subjects. These provisions extend to include liabilities or compensation to the subject's dependents. (Consult the documentation of an appropriate ethics research committee for further information.)

Self-consciousness   Self-conscious concerns being overly aware of one's own actions or states. This may involve being intensely aware of oneself in an essentially "positive" perspective. Alternatively, self-conscious may involve being ill-at-ease, because the individual is uncomfortably aware that he or she is the object of observation by others. Concerning ethical decision making, an individual, may experience both "positive" and "negative" forms of self-consciousness. (See any standard or medical dictionary for additional definitions and information.)

Virtue Ethics   A traditional ethical theory that "claims that most ethicists go wrong in seeking rules to govern particular actions" (see Kuczewski, 2000, [On-line] for additional information). Kuczewski goes on to say:

> Particular actions are so variable that they require a good deal of judgement, not inflexible rules. Thus, the virtue ethicist asks what kind of character traits we should develop in order to become the kind of persons who will judge well in these variable situations. This line of thought is usually associated with Aristotle and Thomas Aquinas but has many capable contemporary exponents, in bioethics as well as general ethics. [On-line]

Zero Reject Principle   This principle concerns the assurance of services to all children with disabilities. Usually, the development of the principle relates to a response of a legislative body to a court decision concerning the provision of educational services. By extension, when there is zero reject principle legislation educational authorities must also actively try to find all children with disabilities in their jurisdictions. (See Jacob-Timm & Hartshorne, 1994, pp. 99–100 for additional information.)

REFERENCES

Beauchamp, T., & Childress, J. (1994). *Principles of biomedical ethics* (4th ed.). New York: Oxford University Press.

Creaser, B., & Dau, E. (Eds.). (1996). The anti-bias approach in early childhood. Pymble, NSW: HarperEducationalPublishers.

Emanuel, E. J. (1991). *The ends of human life: Medical ethics in a liberal polity.* Cambridge, MA: Harvard University Press.

Hallahan, D. P., & Kauffman, J. M. (1991). *Exceptional children: Introduction to special education* (5th ed.). Englewood Cliffs, NJ: Prentice-Hall.

Hardman, M. L., Drew, C. J., Egan, M. W., & Wolf, B. (1993). *Human exceptionality: Society, society, and family* (4th ed.). Boston: Allyn & Bacon.

Jacob-Timm, S., & Hartshorne, T. (1994). *Ethics and law for school psychologists* (2nd ed.). Brandon, VT: Clinical Psychology Publishing.

Jonsen, A. R. (1991). Casuistry as methodology in clinical ethics. *Theoretical Medicine, 12*(4), 295–307.

Kagan, S. (1989). *The limits of morality.* New York: Oxford University Press.

Kant, I. (1996). *Critique of practical reason.* (T. K. Abbott, Trans.). Amherst: Prometheus Books. (Original work published 1909)

Keeves, J. P. (Ed.). (1997). *Educational research, methodology, and measurement: An international handbook* (2nd ed.). Oxford: Elsevier Science.

Keith-Spiegel, P., & Koocher, G. P. (1985). *Ethics in psychology.* New York: Oxford University Press.

Kuczewski, M. (2000). *Thinking about ethics. Introduction: Method in bioethics* [On-line]. Available: http://www-hsc.usc.edu/~mbernste/THINKINGABOUTETHICS.HTML

Merriam-Webster's *New collegiate dictionary* (10th ed.). (1999). Springfield, MA: Merriam-Webster.

Mosby's medical, nursing, and allied health dictionary (3rd ed.). (1990). St. Louis: C. V. Mosby.

Northern, J. L., & Downs, M. P. (1984). *Hearing in children* (3rd ed.). Baltimore: Williams & Wilkins.

Parashar, O. M. (1977). *Dictionary of special education.* Freeport, NY: Educational Activities.

Rawls, J. (1971). *A theory of justice.* Cambridge, MA: Harvard University Press.

Reynolds, C. R., & Fletcher-Janzen, E. (Eds.). (1990). *Concise encyclopedia of special education.* New York: John Wiley & Sons.

Roeher Institute. (1999). *Genome(s) and justice: Reflections on a holistic approach to genetic research, technology and disability.* Toronto: Roeher Institute/Inclusion International.

Smith, D. D., Luckasson, R., & Crealock, C. (1995). *Introduction to special education in Canada: Teaching in an age of challenge.* Scarborough, ON: Allyn & Bacon.

Snoddon, K. (2000). Genetics: Genetics and Deaf people. In C. Aquiline (Ed.) *World Federation of the Deaf: News, 13*(1), 5–6.

Strong, C. (1988). Justification in ethics. In B. Brody (Ed.), *Moral theory and moral judgments in medical ethics* (pp. 193–211). Dordrecht: Kluwer Academic.

Tri-Council Working Group. (1996). *Code of conduct for research involving humans.* Ottawa, ON: Minister of Supply and Services.

Turkington, C., & Sussman, A. E. (1992). *The encyclopedia of deafness and hearing disorders.* New York: Facts On File.

Williams, P. (1991). *The special education handbook: An introductory reference.* Milton Keynes, UK: Open University Press.

Wolff-Heller, K., Alberto, P. A., Forney, P. E., & Schwartzman, M. N. (1996). *Understanding physical, sensory, and health impairments: Characteristics and educational implications.* Pacific Grove, CA: Brooks/Cole.

World Federation of the Deaf (WFD) WFD News (May 2000). Principles for genetic research (p. 6). Excerpted from "Genome(s) and Justice: Reflections on a Holistic Approach to Genetic Research, Technology and Disability," the Roeher Institute in Cooperation with Inclusion International. I'Instute Roeher Institute, 1999. *World Federation of the Deaf: News, 13*(1), 6.

REFERENCES

Alexander, F. K. (1998). Vouchers in American education: Hard legal and policy lessons from higher education. *Journal of Education Finance, 24*(2), 153–178.

American Speech-Language-Hearing Association. (1995). Code of Ethics of the American Speech-Language-Hearing Association (1992). In F. H. Silverman, *Speech, language, and hearing disorders* (pp. 228–238). Boston: Allyn & Bacon.

Annison, J., Jenkinson, J., Sparrow, W., & Bethune, E. (1995). *Disability: A guide for health professionals.* Melbourne: Thomas Nelson.

Antia, S. (1998). School and classroom characteristics that facilitate the social integration of Deaf and hard of hearing children. In A. Weisel (Ed.), *Issues unresolved: New perspectives on language and deaf education* (pp. 148–160). Washington DC: Gallaudet University Press.

Archibald, S. (2000). *Cochlear implantation in children—Influencing educational choices?* Plennary at the 19th International Congress on Education of the Deaf and 7th Asia-Pacific Congress on Deafness (July, 11). Sydney, Australia.

Arras, J. (1994). The role of cases in bioethics. *Indiana Law Journal, 69,* 983–1013.

Arras, J. (1997). Nice story, but so what? In H. Lindemann-Nelson (Ed.), *Stories and their limits* (pp. 65–88). New York: Routledge.

Australian Association of the Deaf. (n.d.). *Policy on the cochlear implant.* Petersham: Australian Association of the Deaf.

Bacharach, S. B. (1990). Putting it all together—educational reform: Making sense of it all. In S. B. Bachrach (Ed.), *Educational reform—making sense of it all* (pp. 415–430). Boston: Allyn & Bacon.

Balkany, T., Hodges, A. V., & Luntz, M. (1996). Update on cochlear implantation. *Otolaryngol-Clin-North America, 29*(2), 277–289.

Banks, T. (1999, June). A stitch in time: Organizations would do well to do good right now as ethics-to-go might give you heartburn. *Management Today,* 14–19.

Barton, K. (1995). Disability: An issue for sociological analysis. In R. Kahane (Ed.), *Educational advancement and distributive justice—between equality and equity* (pp. 326–340). Jerusalem: Magnes Press.

Bat-Chava, Y. (1993), Antecedents of self-esteem of deaf people: A meta-analitic review. *Rehabilitation Psychology, 38*(4), 221–234.

Beauchamp, T. L. (1994). Principles and other emerging paradigms in bioethics. *Indiana Law Journal, 69,* 955–971.

Beauchamp, T. L., & Childress, J. F. (1989). *Principles of biomedical ethics* (3rd ed.). New York: Oxford University Press.

Beauchamp, T. L., & Childress, J. F. (1994). *Principles of biomedical ethics* (4th ed.). New York: Oxford University Press.

Beaver, D. L., Hayes, P. L., & Luetke-Stahlman, B. (1995). In-service trends: General education on teachers working with educational interpreters. *American Annals of the Deaf, 140*(1), 38–42.

Bell, R., & Pitt, D. (1976). The case of Mackenzie. In R. Bell, D. Pitt, & M. Skilbeck (Eds.), *The scope of curriculum study* (pp. 7–44). Milton Keynes: The Open University Press.

Bertling, T. (1994). *A child sacrificed to the deaf culture.* Wilsonville, OR: Kodiak Media Group.

Blume, S. (1997). The rhetoric and counter rhetoric of a "Bionic Technology." *Science, Technology and Human Values, 22*(1), 31–56.

Brady, L. (1990). *Curriculum development* (3rd ed.). Sydney: Prentice-Hall.

British Deaf Association (BDA). (1996). *The right to be equal: The British Deaf Association Education Policy.* London: British Deaf Association.

Bull, B. L. (1983). Ethics in the preservice curriculum. In K. A. Strike & P. L. Ternasky (Eds.), *Ethics for professionals in education: Perspectives for preparation and practice* (pp. 69–83). New York: Teachers College.

Bunch, G. O. (1987). *The curriculum and the hearing-impaired student.* Boston: Little Brown and Company.

Bunch, G. (1994). An interpretation of full inclusion. *American Annals of the Deaf, 139*(2), 150–152.

Calderon, R., & Green, M. T. (1999). Stress and coping in hearing mothers of children with hearing loss: Factors affecting mother and child adjustment. *American Annals of the Deaf, 44*(2), 7–17.

Canadian Psychological Association. (1999). *Canadian Code of Ethics for Psychologists—Revised 1991* [On-line]. Available: http://www.cpa.ca:80/ethics.html.

Chen, M. (1997). School choice as a bargain in a sectarian educational system. In R. Shapira & P. W. Cookson, Jr. (Eds.), *Autonomy and choice in context: An international perspective* (pp. 41–76). New York: Pergamon.

Christie, R. J., & Hoffmaster, C. B. (1986). *Ethical issues in family medicine.* Oxford: Oxford University Press.

Chubb, J. E., & Moe, T. M. (1990). *Politics, markets, and America's schools.* Washington DC: The Brookings Institution.

Chubb, J. E., & Moe, T. M. (1997). Politics, markets, and equality in schools. In R. Shapira & P. W. Cookson, Jr. (Eds.), *Autonomy and choice in context: An international perspective* (pp. 203–248). New York: Pergamon.

Cibinel, A., & Kiwanuka, J. (1998). *Human rights and disabled people.* Paper presented at UN Human Rights Vienna Conference, June 1998.

Claydon, L., Knight, T., & Rado, M. (1977). *Curriculum and culture: Schooling in a pluralist society.* Sydney: Allen & Unwin.

Cocks, E., & Stehlik, D. (1995). History of services. In J. Annison, J. Jenkinson, W. Sparrow, & E. Bethune (Eds.), *Disability: A guide for health professionals* (pp. 8–30). Melbourne: Thomas Nelson.

Conway, R., Bergin, L., & Thornton, K. (1996). *Abuse and adults with intellectual disability living in residential services.* Mawson, National Council on Intellectual Disability.

Council for Exceptional Children (CEC). (1997). *CEC Code of Ethics and Standards of Practice (1997)* [On-line]. Available: http://www.cec.sped.org/ps/code.htm.

Creaser, B., & Dau, E. (Eds.). (1996). *The anti-bias approach in early childhood.* Pymble, NSW: HarperEducationalPublishers.

Crouch, R. A. (1997). Letting the deaf be Deaf. Reconsidering the use of cochlear implants in prelingually deaf children. *Hastings Center Report, 27*(4), 14–21.

Cued Speech. (2000). *Information sheet.* Cued Speech Association.

Darrow, M. (1996). International Human Rights Law and Disability: Time for an International Convention on the Human Rights of People with Disabilities. *Australian Journal of Human Rights, 3*(1), 69–96.

Davila, R. (2000). *Education of the Deaf in the new millennium: Assessing the past and projecting into the future.* Keynote Address, International Congress on Education of the Deaf. Sydney: The Australian Association of Teachers of the Deaf.

Davis, L. J. (1995). *Enforcing normalcy: Disability, deafness, and the body.* New York: Verso.

Deacon, J. J. (1974). *Tongue tied.* New York: Scribner.

Deafax Trust. (2000). *Deafchild International.* Presentation at the 19th International Congress on the Education of the Deaf, Sydney, July 2000.

DELTA. (1999). *DELTA's Education Policy: The right to be heard.* DETLA.

De Matteo, A. J., Lou, M. W., & Burke, F. (1990). *The impact of deafness on development.* Paper presented at Grand Rounds, Department of Psychiatry, University of California San Francisco.

Dunn, L. M. (1968). Special education for the mildly retarded—Is much of it justifiable? *Exceptional Children, 35,* 5–22.

Eatough, M. (2000, May). Deaf children and teachers of the deaf, Raw data from the BATOD Survey 1998. *BATOD magazine.*

Education Department of Victoria. (1985). *Curriculum Frameworks P-12: An introduction.* Melbourne: Author.

Emanuel, E. J. (1991). *The ends of human life: Medical ethics in a liberal polity.* Cambridge, MA: Harvard University Press.

Encyclopedia Britannica. (2000). *Ethics* [On-line]. Available: (http://www.britannica.com).

Encyclopedia Britannica. (2000). *Human rights* [On-line]. Available: (http://www.britannica.com).

Estabrooks, W. (Ed.). (1994). *Auditory-verbal therapy for parents and professionals.* Washington, DC: Alexander Graham Bell Association for the Deaf.

Farrell, P. M., & Fost, N. C. (1989). Long-term mechanical ventilation in pediatric respiratory failure: Medical and ethical considerations. *American Review of Respiratory Disease, 140,* S36–S40.

Fine, M., & Asch, A. (Eds.). (1988). *Women with disabilities: Essays in psychology, culture and politics* (Health, Society and Policy Series). Philadelphia: Temple University Press.

Fletcher, A. (1995). *Information kit on the United Nations standard rules for the equalization of opportunities for persons with disabilities.* London: Disability Awareness in Action.

FNDC Newsletter. (1999). Your rights as a parent. In B. Penman, *Children with a hearing loss: Parents rights* [On-line]. Found on:http://www.brandysign.com/rights.html.

Fortnum, H., Davis, A., Butler, A., & Stevens, J. (1996). *Health service implications of changes in aetiology and referral patterns of hearing impaired children in Trent 1985–1993. Report to Trent Health.* Nottingham and Sheffield: MRC Institute of Hearing Research and Trent Health.

Foster, S. (1989). Reflections of a group of deaf adults on their experiences in mainstream and residential school programs in the United States. *Disability, Handicap and Society, 4,* 37–56.

Fox, J. (1999). Sending public school students to private schools. *Policy Review, 93,* 25–29.

Frank, A. W. (1997). *The wounded storyteller: Body, illness, and ethics.* Chicago: University of Chicago Press.

Frankena, W. K. (1973). *Ethics* (2nd ed.). Englewood Cliffs, NJ: Prentice-Hall.

Fulcher, G. (1989). *Disabling policies? A comparative approach to education policy and disability.* London: The Falmer Press.

Gabbard, S. A., Thompson, V., & Brown, M. A. (1998, December). Considerations for newborn hearing screening, audiological assessment and intervention. *Audiology Today.*

Gal, N. (1995). *The individual, the authority and the letter of the law—The Israeli supreme court's position on parent's choice of school.* Jerusalem: Research Institute for Innovation in Education, School of Education, the Hebrew University in Jerusalem. (In Hebrew.)

Geers, A., & Moog, M. S. (Eds.). (1994). Effectivenesss of cochlear implants and tactile aids for deaf children: The sensory aids study at Central Institute for the Deaf. *The Volta Review, 96*(5), 1–231.

Glascock, P. C., Robertson, M., & Coleman, C. (1997). *Charter schools: A review of literature and an assessment of perception.* Paper presented the Annual Conference of Mid-South Educational Research Association. Memphis, TN.

Glassner, B. (1992). *Bodies: The tyranny of perfection.* Los Angeles: Lowell House.

Goldring, E., Hawley, W., Saffold, R., & Smrekar, C. (1997). Parental choice: Consequences for students, families and schools. In R. Shapira & P. W. Cookson, Jr. (Eds.), *Autonomy and choice in context: An international perspective* (pp. 353–388). New York: Pergamon.

Goldstein, H., & Schein, J. D. (1964). Factors in the definition of deafness as they relate to incidence and prevalence. *Proceedings of the Conference on the Collection of Statistics of Severe Hearing Impairments and Deafness in the United States. March 19–20, 1964.* Public Health Service Publication No. 1227. Washington, DC: USGPO.

Gooding, C. (1994). *Disabling laws. Enabling acts: Disability rights in Britain and America.* London: Pluto Books.

Gorney, D. J., & Yesseldyke, J. E. (1992). *Students with disabilities use of various options to access alternative schools and learning centers.* Research Report No. 3. Enrollment options for students with disabilities. University of Minnesota, Minneapolis.

Gregory, S., & Hartley, G. (Eds.). (1991). *Constructing deafness.* London: Pinter.

Grosjean, F. (1992). The bilingual and the bicultural person in the hearing and in the Deaf world. *Sign Language Studies, 77,* 307–320.

Gross, N. E. (1985). *Everyone here spoke sign language: Hereditary deafness on Martha's Vineyard.* Cambridge, MA: Harvard University Press.

Hallahan, D. P., & Kauffman, J. M. (1991). *Exceptional children: Introduction to special education* (5th ed.). Englewood Cliffs, NJ: Prentice-Hall.

Hardman, M. L., Drew, C. J., Egan, M. W., & Wolf, B. (1993). *Human exceptionality: Society, society, and family* (4th ed.). Boston: Allyn & Bacon.

Harris, G. A. (1983). *Broken ears, wounded heart.* Washington, DC: Gallaudet College Press.

Hellman, S. A., Chute, P. M., Kretchmer, R. E., Nevins, M. E., Parisier, S. C., & Thurston, L. C. (1991). The development of the Children's Implant Profile. *American Annals of the Deaf/Reference, 136*(2), 77–81.

Henderson, D., & Hendershott, A. (1991). ASL and the family system. *American Annals of the Deaf, 136,* 325–329.

Henderson, R. A. (1995). Worldwide school reform movements and students with disabilities. *British Journal of Special Education, 22*(4) 148–151.

Higgins, P., & Nash, J. (Eds.). (1987). *Understanding deafness socially.* Springfield, IL: C. C. Thomas.

Hillyer, B. (1993). *Feminism and disability.* Norman, OK: University of Oklahoma Press.

Hoffmaster, B. (1990). Morality and the social sciences. In G. Weisz (Ed.), *Social science perspectives on medical ethics* (pp. 241–260). Boston: Kluwer Academic.

Hoffmaster, B. (1992). Can ethnography save the life of medical ethics? *Social Science and Medicine, 35*(12), 1421–1431.

Hoffmaster, B. (1994). The forms and limits of medical ethics. *Social science and medicine, 39*(9), 1155–1166.

Hughes, B. (2000). Medicine and the aesthetic invalidation of disabled people. *Disability & Society, 15,* 555–568.

Hyde, M., & Power, D. (2000). Informed parental consent for cochlear implantation of young deaf children: Social and other considerations in the use of the "Bionic Ear." *Australian Journal of Social Issues, 35,* 117–128.

Inbar, D. (1994a). Choice in education in Israel. In D. Inbar (Ed.). *Choice in education in Israel—concepts, approaches and attitudes* (pp. 2–11). Jerusalem: The Ministry of Education. (In Hebrew.)

Jackson, P. W. (1968). *Life in classrooms.* New York: Holt, Rinehart and Winston.

Jacobs, L. M. (1989). *A deaf adult speaks out* (3rd ed.). Washington, DC: Gallaudet University Press.

Jacob-Timm, S., & Hartshorne, T. (1994). *Ethics and law for school psychologists* (2nd ed.). Brandon, VT: Clinical Psychology Publishing.

Jennings, B. (1990). Ethics and ethnography in neonatal intensive care. In G. Weisz (Ed.), *Social science perspectives on medical ethics* (pp. 261–272). Boston: Kluwer Academic.

Jimerson, L. (1998). *Hidden consequences of school choice: Impact on programs, finances and accountability.* Paper presented at the Annual Meeting of the American Educational Research Association. San Diego, CA.

Johnson, P. (1991). *The birth of the modern.* New York: HarperCollins.

Johnson, R. C. (2000). *Gallaudet forum addresses cochlear implant issues. Research at Gallaudet, Spring 2000.* Washington, DC: Gallaudet University, Gallaudet Research Institute.

Jonsen, A. R. (1991). Casuistry as methodology in clinical ethics. *Theoretical Medicine, 12*(4), 295–307.

Jonsen, A. R., Siegler, M., & Winslade, W. (1992). *Clinical ethics.* New York: McGraw-Hill.

Kagan, S. (1989). *The limits of morality.* New York: Oxford University Press.

Kant, I. (1996). *Critique of practical reason.* (T. K. Abbott, Trans.). Amherst: Prometheus Books. (Original work published 1909.)

Karchmer, M. A. (1985). A demographic perspective. In E. Cherow, N. Matkin, & R. Trybus (Eds.), *Hearing impaired children and youth with developmental disabilities: An interdisciplinary foundation for service* (pp. 36–56). Washington, DC: Gallaudet College Press.

Keeves, J. P. (Ed.). (1997). *Educational research, methodology, and measurement: An international handbook* (2nd ed.). Oxford: Elsevier Science.

Keith-Spiegel, P., & Koocher, G. P. (1995). *Ethics in psychology.* New York: Oxford University Press.

Kelley, P., & Gale, G. (1998). *Towards excellence: Effective education for students with vision impairments.* North Rocks, NSW: North Rocks Press.

Kuczewski, M. (2000). *Thinking about ethics. Introduction: Method in bioethics* [On-line]. http://www-hsc.usc.edu/~mbernste/THINKINGABOUTETHICS.HTML.

Kuhse, H. (1987). *The sanctity-of-life doctrine in medicine: A critique.* Oxford: Clarendon Press.

Kuhse, H. (1995). Quality of life as a decision-making criterion. In A. Goldsworth, W. Silverman, D. K. Stevenson, E. W. D. Young, & R. Rivers (Eds.), *Ethics and perinatology.* New York: Oxford University Press.

Kuhse, H., & Singer, P. (1985). *Should the baby live? The problem of handicapped infants.* Oxford: Oxford University Press.

Ladd, J. (1980). The quest for a code of professional ethics: An intellectual and moral confusion, In R. Chalk, M. S. Frankel, & S. B. Chafer (Eds.), *AAAS professional ethics project: Professional ethics activities in the scientific and engineering societies* (pp. 154–159). Washington, DC: American Association for the Advancement of Science.

Levine, E. S. (1960). *The psychology of deafness.* New York: Columbia University Press.

Lewis, S. (1999). Educational routes-ways, and means. In J. Stokes (Ed.), *Hearing impaired infants: Support in the first eighteen months* (pp. 163–191). London: Whurr.

Lewis, S., & Hostler, M. (1998). *Some outcomes of mainstream education.* London: Ewing Foundation.

Lindemann-Nelson, H. (1997). *Stories and their limits.* New York: Routledge.

Lindemann-Nelson, H., & Lindemann-Nelson, J. (1995). *The patient in the family.* New York: Routledge.

Luetke-Stahlman, B., (1992). Comparing four input models of parental questions to hearing and deaf preschoolers. *ACEHI Journal, 18*(2/3), 93–101.

Lynas, W. (1999). Communication options. In J. Stokes (Ed.). *Hearing impaired infants: Support in the first eighteen months* (pp. 98–128). London: Whurr.

Lynas, W., Lewis, S., & Hopwood, V. (1997). Supporting the education of deaf children in mainstream schools. *Journal British Association of Teachers of the Deaf, 21*(2), 41–45.

Mabbott, J. D. (1966). *An introduction to ethics.* London: Hutchinson University Library.

Marschark, M. (1997). *Raising and educating a deaf child.* New York: Oxford University Press.

Marzella, P. L., & Clark, G. M. (1999). Growth factors, auditory neurones and cochlear implants: A review. *Acta Oto-Laryngologica, 119,* 407–412.

McCracken, W., & Sutherland, H. (1981). *Deafability not disability.* Clevedon, UK: Multilingual Matters.

McGroarty, D. (1996). Bus ride to nowhere. *American Enterprise, 7*(5), 38–41.

Meekosha, A. (1999). *Disability and human rights. Attorney General's Forum on Domestic Human Rights.* Canberra, ACT: Office of the Attorney General.

Merriam-Webster's collegiate dictionary (10th ed.). (1999). Springfield, MA: Merriam-Webster.

Messick, S. (1989). Validity. In R. Linn (Ed.), *Educational measurement* (3rd ed), (pp. 13–103). New York: American Council on Education and Macmillan Publishing Company.

Meyerson, A. (1999). A model of cultural leadership: The achievements of privately funded vouchers. *Policy Review, 93,* 20–24.

Miner, I. D. (1996). Ethics of cochlear implantation [letter]. *Otolaryngol-Head-Neck Surgery, 115*(6), 584–585.

Moores, D. F. (1990). Research in educational aspects of deafness. In D. F. Moores & K. P. Meadow-Orlans (Eds.), *Educational and developmental aspects of deafness* (pp. 11–24). Washington, DC: Gallaudet University Press.

Moores, D. F. (1996). *Educating the deaf: Psychology, principles, and practices* (4th ed.). Boston: Houghton Mifflin.

Moores, D. F. (2001). *Educating the deaf: Psychology, principles, and practices* (5th ed.). Boston: Houghton Mifflin.

Morris, D. W. H. (1992). *Dictionary of communication disorders* (2nd ed.). London: Whurr.

Morse, J. M., & Field, P. A. (1995). *Qualitative research methods for health professionals.* Thousand Oaks, CA: Sage.

Moseby's medical, nursing, and allied health dictionary (3rd ed.). (1990). St. Louis: C. V. Mosby.

Morse, J. M., & Field, P. A. (1995). *Qualitative research methods for health professionals.* Thousand Oaks, CA: Sage.

Muirhead, E. S., James, P. L., & Griener, G. G. (1995). Clinical ethics forum: An examination of principle-centered decision-making in human communication disorders. *Journal of Speech-Language Pathology and Audiology, 19*(3), 187–196.

Müller-Hill, B. (1994). Lessons from a dark and distant past. In A. Clarke (Ed.), *Genetic counselling: Practice and principles* (pp. 133–141). London: Routledge.

Murray, T. (1997). What do we mean by 'narrative ethics'? In H. Lindemann-Nelson (Ed.), *Stories and their limits* (pp. 3–17). New York: Routledge.

Nathan, J. (1997). Possibilities, problems, and progress: Early lessons from the charter movement. In R. Shapira & P. W. Cookson, Jr. (Eds.), *Autonomy and choice in context: An international perspective* (pp. 389–405). New York: Pergamon.

National Association of the Deaf. (2000). *NAD interpreter code of ethics* [On-line]. Available: http://nad.policy.net/proactive/newsroom/release.vtml?id=17200.

National Association of the Deaf. (2000). *NAD position statement on cochlear implants* [On-line]. Available: http://www.nad.org/infocenter/newsroom/papers/CochlearImplants.html.

National Deaf Children's Society. (1996). *Quality standards in pediatric audiology, Vol. 2.* London, NDCS.

Newell, C. (1991). A critical evaluation of the NH & MRC's "The Ethics of Limiting Life—Sustaining Treatment" and related perspectives of bioethics of disability. *Australian Disability Review, 4,* 46–57.

Nix, G. W. (Ed.). (1977). The rights of hearing-impaired children. *The Volta Review, 79*(5), 263–351.

Noble, K. A. (1995). *The international education quotations encyclopedia.* Buckingham: Open University Press.

Northern, J. L., & Downs, M. P. (1984). *Hearing in children* (3rd ed.). Baltimore: Williams & Wilkins.

NSW Office of Disability. (1994). *Disability Services Act 1993 Statement of Principles.* Sydney: Government of New South Wales. Social Policy Directorate.

Oliver, M. (1996). *Understanding disability: From theory to practice.* New York: St. Martin's.

Owens, R. E., Jr. (1996). *Language development: An introduction* (4th ed.). Needham Heights, MA: Macmillan.

Oxford dictionary (the concise) (8th ed.). (1991) Oxford: Clarendon.

Padden, C., & Humphries, T. (1988). *Deaf in America: Voices from a culture.* Cambridge, MA: Harvard University Press.

Parashar, O. M. (1977). *Dictionary of special education.* Freeport, NY: Educational Activities.

Parasnis, I., Davila, R. R., Leslie, P., Weisel, A., Matsufigi, M., & Storbeck, C. (2000). *Multicultural perspectives on inclusion and access issue in deaf education.* Panel at the 19th International Congress on Education of the Deaf and 7th Asia-Pacific Congress on Deafness (July 12). Sydney, Australia.

Parens, E., & Asch, A. (1999). The disability rights critique of prenatal genetic testing: Reflections and recommendations. *Hastings Center Report, September–October,* Special Supplement.

Parsons, E., & Bradley, D. (1994). Ethical issues in newborn screening for Duchenne muscular dystrophy: The question of informed consent. In A. Clarke (Ed.), *Genetic counselling: Practice and principles* (pp. 95–112). London: Routledge.

Patton, M. (1990). *Qualitative evaluation and research methods* (2nd ed.). Newbury Park, CA: Sage.

Paul, P. V., & Quigley, S. P. (1990). *Education and deafness.* New York: Longman.

Paulette, L. (1993). A choice for K'aila. *Humane Medicine, 9*(1), 13–17.

Pijil, S., & Dyson, A. (1998). Funding special education: A three country study of demand oriented models. *Comparative Education, 34*(3), 61–79.

Pollard, R. Q., Jr. (1996). Conceptualizing and conducting preoperative psychological assessments of cochlear implant candidates. *Journal of Deaf Studies and Deaf Education, 1*(1), 16–28.

Power, D. (1990). Hearing impairment. In A. Ashman, & J. Elkins (Eds.), *Educating children with special needs* (pp. 276–312). Sydney: Prentice-Hall.

Power, D. (1992). Deaf people: A linguistic and cultural minority or a disability group? *Australian Disability Review,* 4–92, 43–48.

Power, D. (1997). *Constructing lives: The Deaf experience.* Brisbane, QLD: Griffith University, Faculty of Education.

Power, D. (2000). *Informed parental consent for cochlear implantation of young deaf children— social and other considerations in the use of the "Bionic Ear."* Paper at the 19th International Congress on Education of the Deaf and 7th Asia-Pacific Congress on Deafness (July 12). Sydney, Australia.

Powers, S., Gregory, S., Lynas, W., McCracken, W., Watson, L., Boulton, A., & Harris, D. (1999). *A review of good practice in deaf education.* London: RNID.

Powers, S., Gregory, S., & Thoutenhoofd, E. (1998). *The educational achievements of deaf children.* London: Department of Education and Employment, HMSO.

Pueschel, S. M. (1991). Ethical considerations relating to prenatal diagnosis of fetuses with Down syndrome. *Mental Retardation, 29*(4), 185–190.

Purtilo, R. B. (1988). Ethical issues in teamwork: The context of rehabilitation. *Archives of Physical Medicine and Rehabilitation, 69,* 318–322.

Quartararo, A. T. (1995). The perils of assimilation in modern France: The Deaf community, social status, and education opportunity, 1815–1870. *Journal of Social History, 29*(1), 5–25.

Rachels, J. (1986). *The end of life: Euthanasia and morality.* Oxford: Oxford University Press.

Rainer, J. D., Altshuler, K. Z., Kallman, F. J., & Deming, W. E. (1963). *Family and mental problems in a deaf population.* New York: Department of Medical Genetics, New York State Psychiatric Institute, Columbia University.

Ramsay, M. (1994). Genetic reductionism and medical genetic practice. In A. Clarke (Ed.), *Genetic counselling: Practice and principles* (pp. 241–260). London: Routledge.

Raskind, M. H., & Higgins, E. L. (1995). Reflections on ethics, technology and learning disabilities: Avoiding the consequences of ill-considered actions. *Journal of Learning Disabilities, 28*(7), 425–438.

Rawls, J. (1971). *A theory of justice.* Cambridge, MA: Harvard University Press.

Reagan, T. (1990). Cultural considerations in the education of deaf children. In D. F. Moores & K. P. Meadow-Orlans (Eds.), *Educational and developmental aspects of deafness.* (pp. 73–84). Washington, DC: Gallaudet University Press.

Reay, D., & Ball, S. (1997). "Spoilt for choice": The working classes and educational markets. *Oxford Review of Education.*

Reynolds, C. R., & Fletcher-Janzen, E. (Eds.). (1990). *Concise encyclopedia of special education.* New York: John Wiley & Sons.

Ries, P. W. (1992). Prevalence and characteristics of persons with hearing trouble, 1990–91. *Vital and Health Statistics, Series 10,* No. 103.

Rittenhouse, R. K., & Dancer, J. E. (1992). Educational and legislative issues in students with hearing loss: Inter-disciplinary considerations. *Volta Review, 94*(1), 9–17.

Roeher Institute. (1999). *Genome(s) and justice: Reflections on a holistic approach to genetic research, technology and disability.* Toronto: Roeher Institute/Inclusion International.

Rosen, S. (1997). *A synopsis of the Bill of Rights for deaf and hard of hearing children* [On-line]. Available: http://nad.policy.net/proactive/newsroom/release.vtml?id=17960.

Rothman, D. J. (1991). *Strangers at the bedside: A history of how law and bioethics transformed medical decision making.* New York: BasicBooks.

Sage, D. D., & Burrello, L. C. (1994). *Leadership in educational reform.* Sydney: Paul Brookes.

Schein, J. D. (1964). Factors in the definition of deafness as they relate to incidence and prevalence. In H. Goldstein & J. D. Schein (Eds.), *Proceedings of the Conference on the Collection of Statistics of Severe Hearing Impairments and Deafness in the United States, March 19–20, 1964.* Public Health Service Publication No. 1227. Washington, DC: USGPO.

Schein, J. D. (1968). *The Deaf community.* Washington, DC: Gallaudet College Press.

Schein, J. D. (1973). Hearing disorders. In L. T. Kurland, J. F. Kurtzke, & I. D. Goldberg (Eds.), *Epidemiology of neurologic and sense organ disorders* (pp. 276–304). Vital and Health Statistics Monographs, American Public Health Association. Cambridge: Harvard University Press.

Schein, J. D. (1989). *At home among strangers.* Washington, DC: Gallaudet University Press.

Schein, J. D., Gentile, A., & Haase, K. (1970). Development and evaluation of an expanded hearing loss scale questionnaire. *Vital and Health Statistics, Series 2,* No. 37.

Schildroth, A., & Motto, S. (1994). Inclusion or exclusion? *American Annals of the Deaf, 139*(2), 163–171.

Schmid, H. (1986). The changing role of management in human services organizations. *Human Systems Management, 6,* 71–81.

Schrader, D. E. (1983). Lawrence Kohlberg's approach and the moral education of education professionals. In K. A. Strike & P. L. Ternasky (Eds.), *Ethics for professionals in education: Perspectives for preparation and practice* (pp. 84–101). New York: Teachers College.

Seddon, T. (1983). The hidden curriculum: An overview. *Curriculum Perspectives, 3*(1), 1–6.

Sela, I., & Weisel, A. (1992). *The Deaf community in Israel.* Tel Aviv, Israel: Association of the Deaf in Israel, National Insurance Institute, JDC Israel, Ministry of Labour and Social Affairs.

Shapira, R., Haymann, R., & Shavit, R. (1995). Autonomy as ethos, content as commodity: An Israeli model for controlled choice and autonomous schools. In R. Kahane (Ed.). *Educational advancement and distributive justice—between equality and equity* (pp. 358–374). Jerusalem: The Magnes Press, The Hebrew University.

Sharp, H. M., & Genesen, L. B. (1996). Ethical decision-making in dysphagia management. *American Journal of Speech-Language Pathology, 5*(1), 15–22.

Sherwin, S. (1992). *No longer patient: Feminist ethics and health care.* Philadelphia: Temple University Press.

Sherwin, S. (1998). A relational approach to autonomy in health care. In S. Sherwin, *The politics of women's health: Exploring agency and autonomy.* Philadelphia: The Feminist Health Care Ethics Research Network. Temple University Press.

Shildrick, M. (1997). *Leaky bodies and boundaries: Feminism, postmodernism and (bio)ethics.* London: Routledge.

Shonkoff, J. P., Hauser-Cram, P., Krauss, M., & Upshur, C. (1992). Development of infants with disabilities and their families. *Monographs of the Society for the Research in Child Development, 57*(6 Serial No. 230).

Silverman, F. H. (1995). *Speech, language, and hearing disorders.* Boston: Allyn & Bacon.

Sinclair, L., & Griffiths, M. (1994). Medical genetics and mental handicap. In A. Clarke (Ed.), *Genetic counselling: Practice and principles.* London: Routledge.

Singer, G. H. S., & Powers, L. E. (Eds.). (1993). *Families, disability, and empowerment: Active coping skills and strategies for family interventions.* Baltimore: Paul H. Brookes.

Singer, P. (1981). *The expanding circle: Ethics and sociobiology.* Oxford: Clarendon Press.

Singer, P. (1993). *Practical ethics* (2nd ed.). Cambridge: Cambridge University Press.

Skilbeck, M. (1976). Appendix 2. The curriculum-development process: A model for school use. In D. Lawton, W. Prescott, P. Gammage, J. Greenwald, & H. McMahon (Eds.), *The child, the school, and society* (pp. 141–144). Milton Keynes: The Open University Press.

Smith, D. D., Luckasson, R., & Crealock, C. (1995). *Introduction to special education in Canada: Teaching in an age of challenge.* Scarborough, ON: Allyn & Bacon.

Snoddon, K. (2000). Genetics: Genetics and Deaf people. In C. Aquiline (Ed.), *World Federation of the Deaf: News, 13*(1), 5–6.

Sockett, H. (1976). *Designing the curriculum.* London: Open Books.

Spinrad, L., & Spinrad, T. (1979). *Speaker's lifetime library.* Englewood Cliffs, NJ: Prentice-Hall.

Statistical Abstract of Israel. (1993). Jerusalem: Bureau of Statistics.

Stevens, S. (2000). *Normalization vs pride and self-expression* [On-line]. Available: http://www.clarity-network.com/.

Stewart, D. (1992). Initiating reform in total communication programs. *The Journal of Special Education, 26,* 68–84.

Stewart, D. A., & Kluwin, T. N. (2001). *Teaching deaf children: Content, strategies, and curriculum.* Boston: Allyn & Bacon.

Stinson, M. S., & Lang, H. G. (1994). Full inclusion: A path for integration or isolation? *American Annals of the Deaf, 139*(2), 156–159.

Strauss, A., & Corbin, J. (1998). *Basics of qualitative research: Grounded theory procedures and techniques* (2nd ed.). Thousand Oaks, CA: Sage.

Stredler-Brown, A., & Yoshinago-Itano, C. (1994). F.A.M.I.L.Y. assessment: A multidisciplinary evaluation tool. In J. Rousch & N. D. Matkin (Eds.), *Infants and toddlers with hearing loss: Family-centered assessment and intervention* (pp. 133–161). Baltimore: York.

Strike, K. A. (1983). Teaching ethical reasoning using cases. In K. A. Strike & P. L. Ternasky (Eds.), *Ethics for professionals in education: Perspectives for preparation and practice* (pp. 102–116). New York: Teachers College.

Strong, C. (1988). Justification in ethics. In B. Brody (Ed.), *Moral theory and moral judgments in medical ethics* (pp. 193–211). Dordrecht: Kluwer Academic.

Sutherland, H., & Kyle, J. (1993). *Deaf children at home: Final report.* Bristol, UK: Center for Deaf Studies.

Sutton-Spence, R., & Woll, B. (1999). *The linguistics of British Sign Language: An introduction.* Cambridge: Cambridge University Press.

Sharp, H. M., & Genesen, L. B. (1996). Ethical decision-making in dysphagia management. *American Journal of Speech-Language Pathology, 5*(1), 15–22.

Sherwin, S. (1992). *No longer patient: Feminist ethics and health care.* Philadelphia: Temple University Press.

Sherwin, S. (1998). A relational approach to autonomy in health care. In S. Sherwin, *The politics of women's health: Exploring agency and autonomy*. The Feminist Health Care, Ethics Research Network. Philadelphia: Temple University Press.

Strauss, A., & Corbin, J. (1998). *Basics of qualitative research: Grounded theory procedures and techniques* (2nd ed.). Thousand Oaks, CA: Sage.

Sydney Morning Herald. (2000, February 12). Frank Cicutto Interview. *Sydney Morning Herald*, p. 39.

Teacher Training Agency. (1999). *National specialist educational needs specialist standards*. London: Teacher Training Agency.

Tri-Council Working Group. (1996). *Code of conduct for research involving humans*. Ottawa, ON: Minister of Supply and Services.

Tucker, B. (1998). Deaf culture, cochlear implants, and elective disability. *Hastings Center Report, 28*(4), 6–14.

Tucker, B. P. (1983). *Board of Education of the Hendrick Hudson Central School District v. Rowley:* Utter chaos. *Journal of Law and Education, 12*(2), 235–245.

Turkington, C., & Sussman, A. E. (1992). *The encyclopedia of deafness and hearing disorders*. New York: Facts On File.

Tyler, R. W. (1949). *Basic principles of curriculum and instruction*. Chicago: University of Chicago Press.

Underwood, J. K., & Mead. J. F. (1995). *Legal aspects of special education and pupil services*. Boston: Allyn & Bacon.

UNESCO. (1994). *The Salamanca statement and framework for action on special needs education. World Conference on Special Needs Education: Access and Quality, Salamanca, Spain, June 7–10, 1994*. UNESCO.

UNSECO. (1994a). *The standard rules on the equalization of opportunities for persons with disabilities*. New York: UN Department of Public Information.

United States Bureau of the Census. (1931). *The blind and deaf-mutes in the United States: 1930*. Washington, DC: USGPO.

Van Hasselt, A. (2000). *Cochlear implants in developing countries*. Paper at the 19th International Congress on Education of the Deaf and 7th Asia-Pacific Congress on Deafness (July 11). Sydney, Australia.

Van Hattum, R. J. (1985). *Organization of Speech-Language Services in the Schools: A manual*. Austin, TX: Pro-Ed.

Vehmas, S. (1999). Discriminative assumptions of utilitarian bioethics regarding individuals with intellectual disabilities. *Disability & Society, 14*, 37–52.

Victorian Council of Deaf People. (1991). *Cochlear implant policy*. Melbourne, VIC: Victorian Council of Deaf People.

Vis Dubé, R. (1995). Creating a bilingual environment for children who are deaf. *ACEHI Journal, 21*(1), 62–68.

Waltzman, S. B., & Cohen, N. L. (Eds.). (2000). *Cochlear implants*. New York: Thieme.

Ward, P. R., Tucker, A. M., Tudor, C. A., & Morgan, D. C. (1977). Self-assessment of hearing impairment: Test of the Expanded Hearing Ability Scale Questionnaire on hearing impaired adults in England. *British Journal of Audiology, 11*, 33–39.

Weisel, A. (1989). Educational placement of hearing impaired students as related to family characteristics, students' characteristics, and preschool intervention. *The Journal of Special Education, 23*(3), 303–312.

Weisel, A. (1991). Routes to postsecondary education for hearing impaired students in Israel. In E. G. Wolf-Schein & J. D. Schein (Eds.), *Postsecondary education for deaf students* (pp. 57–65). Edmonton, AB: Educational Psychology, University of Alberta.

Weisel, A. (1998). Unresolved issues in deaf education. In A. Weisel (Ed.), *Issues unresolved: New perspectives on language and deaf education* (pp. xvii-xxii). Washington DC: Gallaudet University Press.

Wildes, K. W. (2000). *Moral acquaintances: Methodology in bioethics*. Notre Dame: University of Notre Dame Press.

Williams, P. (1991). *The special education handbook: An introductory reference.* Milton Keynes, UK: Open University Press.

Williamson, S., & Goswell, J. (1999). *Sound decision: Do children get bionic ears too young? The story* [On-line]. Available: http://abc.net.au/science/slab/cochlear/default.htm.

Willms, J. D., & Chen, M. (1989). The effect of ability grouping on ethnic achievement gap in Israeli elementary schools. *American Journal of Education, 97*(3), 237–257.

Winzer, M. A., (1998). A tale often told: The early progression of special education. *Remedial and Special Education, 19*(4), 212–219.

Wolf, S. M. (Ed.). (1996). *Feminism and bioethics: Beyond reproduction.* New York: Oxford University Press.

Wolfensberger, W. (1975). *Program analysis of service systems* (3rd ed.). Toronto: National Institute on Mental Retardation.

Wolfensberger, W. (1983). *Guidelines for evaluators during a PASS, PASSING, or similar assessment of human service quality.* Downsview, ON: National Institute on Mental Retardation.

Wolfensberger, W. (1992). *A brief introduction to social role valorisation as a high order concept for structuring human services.* Syracuse, NY: Syracuse University Press.

Wolfensberger, W., & Thomas, S. (1998). Review of A. L. Chappell's (1992). Towards a sociological critique of the normalization principle. *International Social Role Valorization Journal, 2*(2), 12–21.

Wolff-Heller, K., Alberto, P. A., Forney, P. E., & Schwartzman, M. N. (1996). *Understanding physical, sensory, and health impairments: Characteristics and educational implications.* Pacific Grove, CA: Brooks/Cole.

Wood, D., Wood, H., Griffiths, A., & Howarth, I. (1986). *Teaching and talking with deaf children.* Chichester: John Wiley & Sons.

World Federation of the Deaf (WFD) WFD News (May 2000). Principles for genetic research (p. 6). Excerpted from "Genome(s) and Justice: Reflections on a Holistic Approach to Genetic Research, Technology and Disability," the Roeher Institute in Cooperation with Inclusion International. I'Instute Roeher Institute, 1999. *World Federation of the Deaf: News, 13*(1), 6.

Yoshinaga-Itano, C. (1998). *Predictors of successful outcome for deaf and hard of hearing infants and toddlers.* Report presented at the NIDCD Advisory Board, NIH, 5-97.

Yoshinaga-Itano, C., Sedey, A., Coulter, D., & Mehl, A. (1998). The language of early and later identified children with hearing loss. *Pediatrics, 102*(5), 1161–1171.

Young, A. (1999). Hearing parents: Adjustment to a deaf child—The impact of a cultural linguistic model of deafness. *Journal of Social Work Practice, 13*(2), 157–176.

INDEX